Understanding Mental Illnesses

Understanding Mental Illnesses

Edited by **John Dalvi**

FOSTER
ACADEMICS

New Jersey

Published by Foster Academics,
61 Van Reypen Street,
Jersey City, NJ 07306, USA
www.fosteracademics.com

Understanding Mental Illnesses
Edited by John Dalvi

International Standard Book Number: 978-1-63242-417-4 (Hardback)

Printed in the United States of America.

Contents

Preface   VII

Part 1   Prediction   1

Chapter 1   **Risk Factors for Delirium in the Acute Stroke**   3
Zikrija Dostović, Dževdet Smajlović,
Ernestina Dostović and Omer Ć. Ibrahimagić

Chapter 2   **Employment and Mental Illness**   15
Mary Ditton

Chapter 3   **Craving and Indicators of Depression
and Anxiety Levels in Different Time Points
of Intensive Alcohol Dependence Treatment**   63
Maja Rus-Makovec

Chapter 4   **Workplace Functional Impairment
Due to Mental Disorders**   81
Charl Els, Diane Kunyk, Harold Hoffman and Adam Wargon

Part 2   Control   111

Chapter 5   **Early Intervention in
Psychiatry Challenges & Opportunities**   113
Mamdouh El-Adl

Chapter 6   **Bibliotherapy for Chinese Patients
with Depression in Rehabilitation**   125
Yang Wang

Chapter 7   **Lost in the Social World:
How Social Cognitive Deficits Affect Social
Functioning of People with Asperger Syndrome**   141
Mónica Figueira, Inmaculada Fuentes and Juan C. Ruiz

Chapter 8   **Suicidal Cut Throat Injuries: Management Modalities**   163
Adeyi A. Adoga

Part 3   **Conclusion – An Attempt at Integrating
Understanding, Predicting, and Controlling**   177

Chapter 9   **Selfhood: A Theory-Derived Relational Model
for Mental Illness and Its Applications**   179
Luciano L'Abate and Mario Cusinato

Permissions

List of Contributors

Preface

Every book is a source of knowledge and this one is no exception. The idea that led to the conceptualization of this book was the fact that the world is advancing rapidly; which makes it crucial to document the progress in every field. I am aware that a lot of data is already available, yet, there is a lot more to learn. Hence, I accepted the responsibility of editing this book and contributing my knowledge to the community.

This book discusses various aspects related to mental illnesses. In this book, the main focus is on the various background factors that govern the understanding of public attitudes, immigration, stigma, and competencies surrounding mental illness. If we really comprehend the characteristics of mental illness, then we should be able to not just anticipate, but perhaps even to master it, irrespective of the form of mental illness in question. Knowing the extent of severity of the illness, will permit us to predict their long-term effects and help in decreasing its consequences and costs to society. The book makes an attempt to integrate theory, research data, and particular ways to deal with mental illness.

While editing this book, I had multiple visions for it. Then I finally narrowed down to make every chapter a sole standing text explaining a particular topic, so that they can be used independently. However, the umbrella subject sinews them into a common theme. This makes the book a unique platform of knowledge.

I would like to give the major credit of this book to the experts from every corner of the world, who took the time to share their expertise with us. Also, I owe the completion of this book to the never-ending support of my family, who supported me throughout the project.

Editor

Part 1

Prediction

Risk Factors for Delirium in the Acute Stroke

Zikrija Dostović[1], Dževdet Smajlović[1],
Ernestina Dostović[2] and Omer Ć. Ibrahimagić[1]
[1]Department of Neurology,
[2]Department of Anaesthesiology and Reanimatology,
University Clinical Center Tuzla, School of Medicine,
University of Tuzla,
Bosnia and Herzegovina

1. Introduction

1.1 Stroke

According to the World Health Organization (WHO), stroke is defined as the sudden development of focal or global symptoms and signs of disturbance of cerebral function lasting more than 24 hours or leading to death, as a result of the pathological processes of vascular origin (Thorvaldsen et al., 1995).

The basic classification of stroke, according to the type of pathological process, is into ischemic stroke, which comprises 70-85%, and hemorrhagic. An ischemic stroke develops due to the inability of supply to brain tissue oxygen and glucose due to occlusion vessel. If the "outbursts" of blood within the brain mass, there is intracerebral hemorrhage, which makes 15-20% of strokes, while the penetration of the blood in the subarachnoid space, usually as a result of aneurysm rupture, leading to a subarachnoid hemorrhage, which makes 5-10% of all strokes.

Stroke leads to focal or multifocal neuropsychological disorders. Given that in clinical stroke in the forefront of motor deficits, disturbance of consciousness and disturbance of speech functions, a very common disorder and the function of other organ systems, most of the neuropsychological symptoms are observed after the acute phase when the general and neurological status stabilized, or when we are able to perform certain neuropsychological tests (Dostović, 2007).

Stroke leads to the different degree of physical, cognitive and psychosocial dysfunctioning. The recovery of patients depends on the severity of disability, the rehabilitation program, but also the subsequent maintenance of achieved function, as well as care and support of family and environment.

1.2 Delirium

According to the International Classification of Diseases and Related Health Problems-Tenth Revision of 1994 delirium, not caused by alcohol or other psychoactive substances, is etiologically nonspecific organic cerebral syndrome, characterized by the simultaneous disturbance of consciousness and attention, perception, thinking, psychomotor behavior,

sense of rhythm of sleep and wakefulness. Running time is different, and the degree ranges from mild to very severe (Anonymous, 1994).
Includes:
- Acute or subacute syndrome of the brain
- Acute or subacute confusing
- Acute or subacute infectious psychosis
- Acute or subacute organic reaction
- Acute or subacute organic psihosindrom
Excludes:
- delirium tremens, caused by alcohol withdrawal state with delirium.

The most important feature of delirium is a disturbance of consciousness accompanied by a change in cognition that can not be better explained by an existing cognitive dysfunction. The disorder develops in a short period of time, usually within hours or days, and tends to fluctuations during the course (Anonymous, 1994).

Delirium is also defined as a transient, essentially reversible dysfunction of brain metabolism, acute or subacute at the beginning of the clinical manifestations, with a wide range of neuropsychological disorders (Wise & Brandt, 1994).

2. Neuropathophysiology of post-stroke delirium

Delirium is one of the most common complications that older patients develop when they are admitted to hospital, affecting up to 30% of all older medical patients (Young & Inouye, 2007). Delirium is a severe, multi-factorial neuropsychiatric disorder with well-defined predisposing and precipitating factors. It is characterised by a disturbance of consciousness and a change in cognition that develop over a short period of time. The mental state characteristically fluctuates during the course of the day, and there is usually evidence from the history, examination or investigations that the delirium is a direct consequence of a medical condition, drug withdrawal or intoxication (Anonymous, 1994). Patients who develop delirium have a high mortality, longer in-patient stay, and higher complication rate, increased risk of institutionalisation and increased risk of dementia (Young & Inouye, 2007; Inouye et al., 1999). Delirium is frequently not recognised by physicians and poorly managed.

Up to one-third of cases of delirium may be preventable. Stroke is a known risk factor for the development of delirium (Ferro et al., 2002). The majority of studies of delirium have reviewed mixed medical, surgical, orthopaedic or ICU patients. There have been only a small number of studies that have assessed delirium post-stroke. These studies have yielded conflicting results and have screened for delirium using different measures at different time intervals.

Although delirium has numerous potential precipitating factors, the clinical presentation is generally similar, suggesting a common pathway in the pathogenesis of delirium. The main cause of delirium is probably disturbance in the neurotransmitter acetylcholine system, particularly in the reticular formation. Reticular formation in the brain stem is the control of attention, sleep and wakefulness.

Knowledge of the pathophysiology of delirium is quite fragmented (White et al., 2002). Delirium is associated with reduction of oxidative metabolism, primarily in the prefrontal areas.

Known anticholinergic drugs or other medications with anticholinergic effects or that bind to muscarinic receptors may also precipitate delirium (Trzepacz et al., 2000). The possibility of delirium was higher in patients taking five or more medications with moderate anticholinergic activity (Lindsesay et al., 2002). Exposure anticholinergic medication was independently and specifically associated with an increase in delirium in elderly patients diagnosed with delirium (Han et al., 2001).

Anticholinesterase activity is increasing in the plasma of patients with delirium. Over the years the loss of cholinergic reserve and focal loss of acetylcholine in the nucleus basalis Meynerti may be the reason that delirium is common in the elderly and patients with dementia. Abnormal termination of the hypothalamic-pituitary-adrenal lines may play a role in the pathophysiology of delirium after acute stroke (Olsson, 1999).

Type II receptors for glucocorticoids, which are present during the high-level (stress) hormones, are heavily expressed in the hippocampus, and intact hipocampal formations, seem to be necessary for adequate negative feedback. Stroke and complications (pain and infection) are stress conditions, the leading to an increase glucocortikoid production, which is not adequately suppressed.

Gustafson et al. (1993) have registered higher corticoid levels and abnormal response to dexamethasone suppression test in patients with acute stroke. Immediately after the stroke, delirium is associated with increased sensitivity to corticoadrenal adrenocorticotropic hormonal stimulation and the decrease in glucocorticoid negative feedback. Corticoids are known to disrupt attention and memory.

Several neurotransmitter systems have been implicated, in particular acetylcholine and dopamine, but also serotonin, noradrenalin and gamma amino butyric acid (GABA). Functional acetylcholine (ACh) deficiency has received most support (Trzepacz , 2000). ACh is involved in several functions that are affected in delirium: arousal, attention, delusions, visual hallucinations, motor activity and memory (Lindsesay et al., 2002). The evidence for ACh involvement in delirium is strong. Anticholinergic drugs can cause delirium in susceptible patients (White, 2002; Lindsesay et al., 2002).

With respect to other neurotransmitter systems, dopamine may also be implicated (Trzepacz, 2000). Dopamine and ACh neurotransmitter systems interact closely and often reciprocally and an imbalance between the two could underlie delirium syndromes. There is evidence that dopamine excess can cause delirium and that dopamine antagonists, particularly neuroleptics, modify the symptoms of delirium (Itil & Fink, 1966). Glucocorticoids are also potentially implicated in delirium; and delirium has been reported in Cushing's syndrome.

Despite being a frequent complication of stroke, the pathophysiology of delirium in the acute stroke is poorly understood. There is no data on how an acute stroke affects neurotransmitter levels in the brain. Drugs with ACh activity are, however, associated with an increased risk of delirium in the acute stroke setting (Caeiro et al., 2004).

Recently, hypoperfusion in the frontal, parietal, and pontine regions have been demonstrated using single photon emission computed tomography (SPECT) scanning in patients with delirium (Fong et al., 2006). It is possible that hypoperfusion, in addition to the acute brain injury, may play an important role in the onset of delirium post-stroke. In addition, one study has found an association between delirium and hypercortisolism in the acute stroke setting (Gustafson, 1993). The pathogenesis of delirium in general remains unknown (White S, 2002).

There are several possible mechanisms for the development of delirium (Table 1).

Mechanism	Example
Altered neurotransmitters	Acetylcholine
	Dopamine
	Serotonin
	Noradrenaline, GABA, glutamate
Altered hypothalamic-pituitary-adrenal axis	Hypercortisolism
Other mechanisms	Cytokine production, e.g. interleukin-1
	Alterations to the blood–brain barrier
	Oxidative stress

Table 1. Possible mechanisms in the development of delirium, (McManus et al., 2007)

It is known that delirium is associated with generalised slowing on electroencephalogram (EEG) that is consistent with widespread cortical dysfunction, which presumably accounts for the wide range of symptoms that delirious patients present with.

3. Risk factors for development of post-stroke delirium

Delirium is a common behavioural disorder in patients with acute stroke (AS). We prospectively analyzed 59 patients with acute stroke in a six-month period in order to determine risk factors for delirium in these patients (Dostović et al., 2009 a,b). For all patients stroke was confirmed by computed tomography within 24 hours after hospitalization. The presence of delirium was assessed according the Delirium Rating Scale R-98 (Trzepac, 1999) and the Diagnostic and Statistical Manual of Mental Disorders - Fourth Edition criteria for delirium (Anonymous, 1994). According to the type of stroke, patients were divided into two groups: with ischemic and hemorrhagic stroke. Laboratory tests were done within the first four days of the stroke onset.
Delirious patients were significantly older (Table 2).

Age and sex	Delirium		Without delirium		Total		p-value
	n	%	n	%	n	%	
Male	25	23.1	83	76.9	108	100.0	
							0.5
Female	34	27.2	91	72.8	125	100.0	
Average age in years	70.0 $\pm$11.3		64.7 $\pm$10.4		66.0 $\pm$10.9		0.001

Table 2. Delirium frequency according to the age and sex

Delirium was more frequent in patients with hemorrhagic stroke (Table 3).

Type of stroke	Delirium		Without delirium		Total		p-value
	n	%	n	%	n	%	
Ischemic	44	22.3	153	77.7	197	100.0	
							0.02
Hemorrhagic	15	41.6	21	58.4	36	100.0	
Total	59	25.3	174	74.7	233	100.0	

Table 3. Delirium frequency according to the type of stroke

In patients with hypertension, delirium was significantly less prevalent (19.3%: 38.3%, p = 0.001), and diabetes had no statistically significant effect on the occurrence of delirium. Patients with delirium had significantly more pronounced leukocytosis, neutrophils, elevated aspartataminotransferasis, sedimentation rate and high temperature (>37.5 C) compared to those without delirium (Table 4).

Biochemical parameters	Delirium n = 59	Without delirium n = 174	p-value
Leucocytes	8.2 (2.9 – 25.5)	6.6 (3.3 – 20)	0.01
Neutrophils	5.7 (1.7 – 13.1)	4.3 (0.5 – 18.9)	0.0001
Triglycerides	1.3 (0.5 – 4.4)	1.6 (0.5 – 7.4)	0.03
AST	28 (7.8 –1008)	24 (11 – 126)	0.002
Potassium	4.0 (2.9 –5.3)	4.1 (3.2 –6.0)	0.04
Increased sedimentation	56 (94.9 %)	146 (83.9%)	0.05
High temperature	34 (57.6 %)	47 (27.0 %)	0.0001

AST – aspartataminotransferaza
Table 4. Biochemical parameters in acute stroke patients

Although stroke is a known predisposing factor for delirium, there have only been a few prospective studies of delirium in the acute stroke setting and these have given conflicting results with prevalence estimates ranging from 13 to 48%. In addition, different independent risk factors for post-stroke delirium have been identified including left-sided strokes, intracerebral haemorrhages, cardioembolic stroke, total anterior circulation infarction, age, neglect, pre-existing cognitive impairment and metabolic disorders post-stroke (Henon, 1999; Sheng, 2006; Dostović, 2007; Dostović et al., 2009 a).

In the one recent study delirium was found in 28% of acute stroke patients. No significant difference was found in the prevalence of delirium between male and female stroke patients. Patients who developed delirium were older than patients who did not. Two models were developed which identified independent determinants of developing delirium including: disphagia on admission, an Barthel score <10, a raised C-reactive protein on admission and poor vision pre-stroke. Pre-stroke cognitive impairment approached statistical significance as an independent predictor of delirium (McManus et al., 2009). These studies used different screening tools and different methodologies. The results of our study are similar to the results of mentioned studies. Precipitating factors for delirium are numerous and generally well recognised (Anonymous, 2006).

There is a predictive model that can identify those patients who will develop delirium after stroke. Apart from the usual predisposing factors, the beginning of delirium after stroke probably dependens on several factors unique to this clinical manifestation: the area of the brain affected by stroke, stroke size, type of stroke, the degree of cerebral hypoperfusion and cerebral edema, and medical complications after stroke.

Gustafson et al. (1991) found that a left-sided stroke is independent risk factors for delirium development. Caeiro et al. (2004) found that delirium was more frequent with hemispherical strokes and after intracerebral haemorrhages. Sheng et al. (2006) found that patients who had a cardioembolic stroke or total anterior circulation infarction (TACI) were more likely to develop delirium. In addition, case reports have suggested that delirium may be associated with specific lesions, for example, in the thalamus and caudate nucleus (Trzepacz, 2000).

| Old age |
| Male gender |
| Dementia |
| Severe illness |
| Visual impairment |
| Psychiatric illness, in particular depression |
| Alcohol excess |
| Physical frailty |
| Polypharmacy |
| Malnutrition |
| Renal impairment |
| Dehydration |

Table 5. Main predisposing factors for development of delirium, (McManus et al., 2007)

Certain types of stroke are more associated with the onset of delirium and complications after a stroke can accelerate the development of delirium. In essence, it is highly likely that the greater stroke cause delirium, but in such patients is increasing and likely to develop medical complications, which in itself can cause delirium. Primary trigger for the start of delirium may be different from case to case.

In patients with stroke, predisposing and precipitating factors for delirium, according to results of other studies are:0 age, extensive motor impairment, paralysis of the left half of the body, pre-existing cognitive decline, metabolic and infectious complications, the right hemisphere cortical lesions, the low score of daily activities, sleep apnea, body mass index less than 27, impaired vision (Gustafson et al., 1991; Henon et al., 1999; Sandberg et al., 2001).

High body temperature, elevated sedimentation rate, hypokalemia, elevated aspartatamniotransferaza, lower triglycerides, neutrophilia, leukocytosis, severe mobility problems, existing chronic diseases, metabolic and infectious complications, older age, a right-hemispheric lesions are possible precipitating factors for the delirium in the acute phase of stroke (Dostović, 2007; Dostović et al., 2009 a,b).

4. Diagnosis, incidence, management and outcome of post-stroke delirium

Delirium is diagnosed and classified according to the cause into: delirium caused by psychoactive substances (during exposure to a substance or during withdrawal), delirium due to general medical condition and vague delirium. The main feature of delirium is a disturbance of consciousness and cognitive functions that occur within a few hours or days, showing a distinct tendency of fluctuation during the day.

At night, the awareness is distinctly worse. A patient with impaired consciousness responds slowly, and its concentration is very difficult. Disturbance of consciousness in terms of disorientation in time and space, and to your self is extremely rare. Memory impairment is usually only for newer content. Speech is often slow and ambiguous and incoherent form of thought.

Behavior may be violent, aggressive and irritable, or passive, slow, docile. Sleep is often disturbed with altered sleep-wake cycle. Delusions may be present, which manifests itself in the form of persecution which are usually transient and not systematized. Disorders of perceptionis most often manifested in the form of illusions, misinterpretations or visual hallucinations. The patient is very terrified. After his recovery he did not remember most events during the episode of delirium.

Delirium is frequently divided into hyperactive, hypoactive, and mixed types. Hyperactive delirium is characterised by increased motor activity with agitated behaviour. Hypoactive delirium is characterised by reduced motor behaviour and lethargy. Although hyperactive delirium has the best prognosis, hypoactive delirium is the most common form of delirium in elderly patients (Anonymous, 2006).

Camus and colleagues (2000) suggested that there are six symptoms suggestive of hypoactive subtype of delirium: lack of facial expression, motor slowing, slowing of speech, and the decrease in reactivity, confusion and mental slowing. Logorea, motor hyperactivity, aggressiveness, stereotype, hyper responsiveness and delusions are symptoms that indicate the hyperactive subtype of delirium.

As stroke is both a recognised predisposing and precipitating factor for delirium, all stroke patients should ideally be screened for delirium on admission and then at regular intervals. The ideal screening tool for the detection of delirium post-stroke would be quick, reliable, evidence-based, accurate, and easy to use by various health professionals, applicable to all stroke patients, able to distinguish between stroke patients with delirium and stroke patients with dementia, depression or psychosis and give an estimate of delirium severity. It should also rely less on level of consciousness, verbal ability and motor disturbance, since these may be independently affected by the cerebral damage secondary to the stroke. Unfortunately, no such tool exists.

Several screening tests for delirium have been developed for use in general hospital settings. No instrument has been specifically designed for the acute stroke setting and there is no consensus on which of the available measures is the best in the acute stroke setting.

The Mini Mental State Examination (MMSE) is a commonly used test to screen for cognitive impairment in routine clinical care. However, the MMSE was not designed to distinguish between delirium and dementia, and patients who were positive for cognitive impairment with the MMSE require further evaluation. The MMSE score is influenced by factors such as language, mood and sensory/motor function which render it unsuitable in the acute stroke setting.

The two most commonly used screening tools for delirium are the Confusion Assessment Method (CAM) (Inouye et al., 1990) and the Delirium Rating Scale (DRS) (Trzepacz, 1988). The CAM was developed in 1990, to be a simple test that general health professionals could use to identify delirium rapidly and accurately. The algorithm was devised from the DSM-III-R criteria for the diagnosis of delirium. Using this algorithm, the diagnosis of delirium is based on four features: acute onset and fluctuating course, and inattention with either disorganised thinking or altered level of consciousness. The CAM has high sensitivity and specificity (0.9) (Inouye et al., 1990). A recent study has highlighted, however, the need for appropriate training if the test is to be performed by nursing staff. The CAM has potential limitations in the acute stroke setting.

Stroke is accompanied with frequent changes in mental state as a result of acute brain lesions, which may contribute to erroneous assessment of the existence of delirium. Also, fluctuations in mental state after a stroke, for example, due to the brain edema can lead us into error in assessing the existence of delirium. Disruption of attention can be difficult to determine in patients with neglect or speech disorders, and assessment of memory disorder after stroke. Disturbance of consciousness is common after stroke and is a consequence of acute brain injury. Thus, while CAM is used frequently in general clinical practice, there is a need for its further validation for the assessment of delirium after acute stroke.

The DRS is a 10-item rating scale, intended for use by medical staff with specific training (Trzepacz et al. 1988). Individual item scores are totalled to generate a 32-point scale. A cut-off of 10 is usually used to diagnose delirium. The DRS allows for estimation of delirium severity. Among the five studies to date on delirium post-stroke, two have used the DRS. One used the DRS alone (Caeiro et al, 2004), the other used the DRS in addition to clinical (DSM-IV) criteria . The DRS and the CAM have been found to have good overall agreement in general medical in-patients (Adamis et al., 2005) but have never been compared in the acute stroke setting. Like the CAM, the DRS has limitations for assessing delirium post-stroke. Pre-stroke cognitive impairment is in itself a risk factor for the development of post-stroke delirium (Fong et al., 2006).

Delirium is a common behavioral disorder after acute stroke. Most studies of postoperative delirium was analyzed and mixed medical geriatric population, and few systematic studies of delirium is specific patients presented with stroke (Gustafson et al., 1991, Gustafson et al. 1993, Henon et al. 1991; Sandberg et al., 2001). Naughton et al. (1997) reported the results of 297 computerized tomographic scan findings in patients with acute delirium; 42 (15%) had one of the acute conditions (stroke, subdural hematoma, tumor). Of the patients with positive computerized tomography, all except two had a disorder of consciousness or new focal neurological deficit. Among the healthy elderly, infection and stroke are the most important etiological factors in delirium. Langhorne et al. (2000) found that the incidence of acute confused state among 311 patients with acute stroke is 36% with weekly prevalence of 24%.

For the purpose of this review, we used the search Pubmed to find all prospective studies of delirium in the acute stroke. The literature is limited; five studies have prospectively studied delirium post-stroke. The total number of patients evaluated in all the studies combined is 804 patients (Gustafson et al., 1991, 1992; Caeiro at al., 2004, Henon et al., 1999, Sheng et al., 2006). In these five studies, the incidence of delirium in the acute phase of stroke varied from 13% to 48% (Table 6).

Due to the specific problems and the complexity of diagnosis and therapy, there are specialized units for care of these patients (Wahlund, Gonzalez, 1999). Among patients with

Study	Gustafson *et al.*	Gustafson *et al.*	Henon *et al.*	Caeiro *et al.*	Sheng *et al.*
Year	1991	1993	1999	2004	2006
Country	Sweden	Sweden	France	Portugal	Australia
Population	Consecutive stroke patients	Consecutive ischaemic stroke patients	Consecutive stroke patients	Consecutive stroke patients	Consecutive stroke patients
Number of patients	145	83	202	218	156
Mean Age (range)	73 (40–101)	75 (44–89)	75 (42–101)	57.3 (24–86)	80 (65–95)
Diagnostic criteria	DSM-III-R	DSM-III-R	DSM-IV and DRS	DRS	DSM-IV
Frequency of assessments	Two assess-ments within first week	Before and after dexamethasone suppression test	Not specified	On admission	Within 3 days of admission
% Delirium	48	42	24	13	25

Table 6. Summary of prospective studies that have assessed post-stroke delirium, (McManus et al., 2007)

delirium in these classes about 40% had dementia, 30% mild cognitive deficit, and 14% depression. It should be keep in mind that the large number of cases of dementia and delirium requires etiological clarification.

Traditionally, delirium has been regarded as having a good prognosis with complete recovery if the underlying cause can be reversed. In addition, delirium was felt to be a short-lived syndrome. Both these assumptions are being increasingly challenged. In studies of patients following hip replacement surgery, delirium is independently associated with poor functional outcome, death and institutionalisation (Marcantonio et al., 2000).

In older patients, delirium is an independent risk factor of sustained poor cognitive and functional status during the year after a medical admission (McCusker et al., 2003). It is also an independent marker for increased mortality at discharge and at 12 months post-discharge, for increased length of stay and institutionalisation (Siddiqi et al., 2006).

There are few data on the outcome of delirium post-stroke, in particular the long-term sequelae. Only one report has 12 months follow-up data (Sheng et al., 2006). The data that are available are summarised in Table 7 and indicate similar prognostic associations to those found in other clinical trials.

Study	Year	Time period	Outcome
Gustafson et al.	1991	Up to discharge	Increased length of stay in patients with delirium (19 versus 13 days, $P<0.001$)
			Increased institutionalisation in patients with delirium (52% of delirious patients institutionalised compared with 15% of non-delirious group)
			Increased need for rehabilitation for delirious patients ($P<0.004$)
			Increased mortality in patients with delirium on admission (11 of 13 deaths occurred in delirium group
Gustafson et al.	1993	Up to discharge	Increased mean length of stay in delirious patients (23.1 versus 15.6 days, $P<0.005$)
			Delirious patients had higher post dexamethasone suppression test cortisol levels ($P<0.001$)
Henon et al.	1998	Up to discharge, in addition 6 month mortality and functional status	Delirious patients had increased length of stay ($P<0.05$), worse functional outcome at discharge ($P<0.001$) and at 6 months ($P<0.001$), lower MMSE score at 6 months ($P<0.002$) but no increase in mortality on discharge ($P = 0.828$) or at 6 months ($P = 0.38$)
Caeiro et al.	2004	Up to discharge	Delirious patients more likely to be dead or dependent ($P = 0.0001$)
Sheng et al.	2006	Up to discharge, 6 and 12 month data on mortality, MMSE, Functional Independence Measure (FIM)	Delirious patients had increased 6 month mortality ($P = 0.02$), increased 12 month mortality ($P = 0.002$) lower MMSEs at 1 month ($P<0.01$) and 12 months ($P<0.01$), lower FIMs at 1, 6 and 12 months ($P<0.01$, $P = 0.003$ and $P = 0.003$ respectively) and increased institutionalisation ($P = 0.002$)

Table 7. Outcome of patients with delirium, (McManus et al., 2007)

Delirium post-stroke is associated with increased length of stay, increased in-patient mortality, increased risk of institutionalisation, increased need for geriatric rehabilitation, increased dependence on discharge and at 6 months, lower MMSE at 6 months and at 12 months, and higher 6 and 12 months mortality rate (Gustafson et al., 1993; Sheng et al., 2006; Henon et al. 1998; Caeiro et al., 2004).

One of the features of delirium is that it is a reversible disorder. In small number of cases is worsening with the development of coma, convulsions and potentially death. Patients may recover completely, to stay with certain consequences, or the recovery of dementia observed that previously existed. In case of patients with various somatic disorders, delirium forecast is largely conditioned by the underlying disease. Elderly patients who develop delirium during hospitalization have a mortality rate of 22% to 76% (Cameron et al., 1987). Increased mortality was documented after discharge from hospital and it was about 25% during the first six months (Trzepacz et al., 1985).

Delirium in patients with stroke is associated with poorer functional but not vital prognosis at discharge and after six months. Patients with stroke and symptoms of delirium have a longer duration of hospital stay and increased incidence of vascular dementia (Gustafson et al., 1991; Henon et al., 1999). Association of delirium with dementia was seen in 8% to 43% depending on the test population (Bucht et al., 1999). In the elderly, mortality due to delirium range from 10% to 75%. In about 20% of patients after cessation of acute confused state, the residues can be identifying up to 6 months later (Hill et al., 1992). These are the most common variety of cognitive deficits. These disorders may be a prelude to the forthcoming dementia. Perhaps that is a critical factor in remaining cognitive reserve. The risk of dementia after delirium in the elderly over 65 years is about 60%, with an annual incidence of 18.1% (Rockvod et al., 1999).

To date, there have been no studies that have evaluated either the prevention or the management of post-stroke delirium. Up to one-third of delirium cases are preventable in medical wards. Inouye et al. (1999) found that a multi-component intervention targeting cognitive impairment, sleep deprivation, immobility, visual and hearing impairment and dehydration reduced the incidence of delirium from 15% in the control group to 9.9% in the intervention group.

With regard to established delirium, the recent guidelines from the Royal College of Physicians give a useful overview of the important aspects of delirium management (Anonymous, 2006). The most important action is the treatment of the underlying cause — this may be the stroke or it may be a complication post-stroke, for example, infection. The patient should be nursed in a good sensory environment and sedation should be used sparingly. Haloperidol is the drug of choice if sedation is needed although the evidence-base for this is weak (Lonergan et al., 2007). Prevention of complications resulting from the onset of delirium — for example, pressure sores and malnutrition — is extremely important. It is entirely conceivable that a multi-component intervention programme that involves training of the stroke unit staff could reduce the incidence of delirium post-stroke and improve the management of established delirium.

5. Conclusion

The main contribution of our research is that we confirm the significance of individual risk factors for delirium after stroke, and previous studies that have been identified and that we have found and new factors not previously been identified. We came to the conclusion that the high body temperature, neutrophilia, leukocytosis, increased sedimentation and aspartatamniotransferasis, previous chronic diseases and older age were possible precipitating factors for delirium in the acute phase of stroke.

Delirium is a common complication after stroke and is independently associated with increased mortality and morbidity. There is a need for more research to clarify the incidence, the predisposing and precipitating factors, and the prognosis in the stroke setting. It seems clear that delirium is a poor prognostic indicator in patients with acute stroke. What is less clear is whether this is because of the underlying stroke type or whether it is by itself an independent marker of poor outcome after stoke. More research is also needed to evaluate preventative and therapeutic strategies in the stroke setting.

It is unclear what the best screening tool is for delirium in the acute stroke setting or how often patients should be screened for delirium. Most screening tools for delirium require a patient who is able to speak. All stroke units should have protocols for screening for delirium, managing patients with established delirium and for preventing delirium in high-risk patients.

6. References

Adamis D, Treloar A, MacDonald A, et al (2005) Concurrent validity of two instruments (the confusion assessment method and the delirium rating scale) in the detection of delirium among older medical patients. *Age Aging* 34: 72-83.

Anonymous (1994) *Diagnostic and statistical Manual of Mental Disorders. 4th ed.* Washington DC: American Psychiatric Association.

Bucht G, Gustafson Y, Sandberg O (1999) Epidemilogy of delirium. *Dement Geriatr Cogn Disord* 10: 315-318.

Caeiro L, Ferro J, Albuquerque R, Figueira ML (2004) Delirium in the first days of acute stroke. *J Neurol* 251: 171-8.

Cameron DJ, Thomas RI, Mulvihill M, Bronheim H (1987) Delirium: a test the Diagnostic and Statistical Manual III criteria on medical inpatients. *J Am Geriatr Soc* 35: 1007-1010.

Camus V, Gonthier R, Dubos G, Schwed P, Simeone I (2000) Etiologic and outcome profiles in hypoactive and hyperactive subtypes of delirium. *J Geriatr Psychiatry* 13: 38-42.

Dostović Z (2007) *Delirium in the acute phase of stroke* (Masters thesis). Faculty of Medicine, University of Tuzla.

Dostović Z, Smajlović D, Sinanović A, Vidovic M (2009) Duration of delirium in the acute stage of stroke. *Acta Clin Croat* 48 (1): 13-17.

Dostović Z, Smajlović D, Sinanović O, Ibrahimagić OĆ, Salihović D, Bećirović E (2009 a) Delirium after stroke. *Acta Med Sal* 38 (1): 26-29.

Ferro JM, Caeiro L, Verdelho A (2002) Delirium in acute stroke. *Curr Opin Neurol* 15: 51-5.

Fong TG, Bogardus ST, Daftary A, et al (2006) Cerebral changes in older patients using 99 m Tc HMPAO SPECT. *J Gerontol A: Biol Sci Med Sci* 61: 1294-9.

Gustafson Y, Olsson T, Erikkson S, Asplund K, Bucht G (1991) Acute confusional states (delirium) in stroke patients. *Cerebrovasc Dis* 1: 257-64.

Gustafson Y, Olsson T, Asplund K, Hagg E (1993) Acute confusional state (delirium) soon after stroke is associated with hypercortisolism. *Cerebrovasc Dis* 3: 33-8.

Han L, McCusker J, Cole M, Abrahamowicz M, Primeau F, Élie M (2001) Use of medications with anticholinergic effects predicts clinical severity of delirium symptoms in older medical patients. *Arch Intern Med* 161: 1099-1105.

Hill CD, Risby E, Morgan N (1992) Cognitive deficits in delirium: assesment over time. *Psychopharmacol Bull* 28: 401-407.

Inouye SK, Bogardus ST, Charpentier PA, et al. (1999)A multicomponent intervention to prevent delirium in hospitalized older patients. *N Engl J Med* 340:669-76.

Langhorne P, Stott DJ, Robertson L (2000) Medical complications after stroke. A multicenter study. *Stroke* 31: 1223-1229.

Lindsesay J, Rockwood K, Macdonald A (2002) *Delirium in Old Age.* Oxford: Oxford University Press Chapter 4.

Lonergan E, Britton A, Lixemberg J et al (2007) Antipsychotics for delirium. *Cochrane Database Syst Rev* 4.

Marcantonio ER, Flacker JM, Michaels M, et al (2000) Delirium is independently associated with poor functional recovery after hip surgery. *J Am Geriatr Soc* 48: 618-24.

McCusker J, Cole M, Dendukuri N, et al (2003) The course of delirium in medical inpatients: a prospective study. *J Gen Intern Med* 18: 696-704.

McManus J, Pathansali R, Stewart R, Macdonald A, Jackson SHJ (2007) Delirium, post-stroke. *Age Ageing* 36: 613-8

McManus J, Pathansali R, Hassan H, Ouldred E, Cooper D, Stewart R, Macdonald A, Jackson S (2009) The course of delirium in acute stroke. *Age Ageing* 38(4): 385-389.

Naughton BJ, Moran M, Ghaly Y, Michalakes C (1997) *Computed tomography scanning and delirium in elder patients* 4: 1107-1110.

National Guidelines, Royal College of Physicians (2006) *The Prevention, Diagnosis and Management of Delirium in Older People.*

Olsson T (1999) Activity in the hypothalamic-pitiutary-adrenal axis and delirium. *Dement Geriatr Cogn Disord* 10: 345-349.

Rockwood K, Cosway S, Carver D, Jarret P, Stadnyk K, Fisk J (1999) The risk of dementia and the death after delirium. *Age Ageing* 28: 551-556.

Sheng AZ, Shen Q, Cordato D, Zhang YY, Kam Yin Chan D (2006) Delirium within three days of stroke in a cohort of elderly patients. *J Am Geriatr Soc* 54: 1192-8.

Sandberg O, Franklin KA, Bucht G, Gustafson Y (2001) Sleep apnea, delirium, depressed mood, cognition and ADL ability after stroke. *J Am Geriatr Soc* 49: 391-397.

Siddiqi N, House AO, Holmes J (2006) Occurrence and outcome of delirium in medical in-patients: a systemic literature review. *Age Aging* 35: 350-64.

Thorvaldsen P, Asplund K, Kuulasma K, Rajakangas A, Schroll M (1995) Stroke incidence, case fatility, and mortality in the WHO MONICA project. *Stroke* 26: 361-367.

Trzepacz P, Teague G, Lipowski Z (1985) Delirium and other organe mental disorders in a general hospital. *Gen Hosp Psychiatry* 7: 101:106.

Trzepacz PT (1999) Update on the neuropathogenesis of delirium. *Dement Geriatr Cogn Disord* 10: 330-334.

Trzepacz PT, Baker RW, Greenhouse J (1988) A symptom rating scale for delirium. *Psychiatry Res* 23: 89-97

Trzepacz PT (2000) Is there a common neural pathway in delirium? Focus on acetylcholine and dopamine. *Semin Clin Neuropsychiatry* 5: 132-148.

Wahlund L-O, Björlin GA (1999) Delirium in clinical practice: expiriences from a specialized delirium ward. *Dement geriatr Cogn Disord* 10: 389-392.

Wise MG, Brandt GT (1994) Delirium. In: Yudofsky SC, Hales RE (eds) *Synopsis of neuropsychiatry*. Washington: American Psychiatric Press.

White S (2002) The neuropathogenesis of delirium. *Rev Clin Gerontol* 12: 62-67.

Young J, Inouye S. (2007) Delirium in the older people. *BMJ* 2007 334: 842-846.

2

Employment and Mental Illness

Mary Ditton
University of New England
Australia

1. Introduction

It is a surprising in some ways that the interaction between employment and mental health or illness has not been subject to greater scrutiny, considering the amount of time the average person spends at work in his lifetime and the risks to mental health that the working environment provides. Probably the stigma of mental illness from the point of view of the employee, and the financial concerns about liability from the point of view of the employer, link together to hinder the exploration of the topic. Nevertheless, contemporary views of health promotion (WHO, 1986) and the Social Determinants of Health (CSDH, 2011)) recognise the impact of employment on health and mental health and various strategies like Health Promoting Workplaces suggest ways of ameliorating the risks and improving employee health overall. It is however necessary to consider a wide definition of employee health to encompass (a) the health of individuals who perform work for a living, (b) the average forty year period of the life span in which employees are in the work environment, (c) the traditional concerns of work related injury but is not restricted to this, and (d) the health promotion aims of quality of life or state of optimum health and striving to reach one's potential. This chapter explores employment and mental illness with this definition of employee health in mind. The main discussion areas are: employment and its link to the burden of mental illness, risks within contemporary employment, and social relationships in the workplace. The key points that will be made are that employment must be considered in the genesis and treatment strategies of mental illness, and that dialogue about mental illness will need to play a greater part in the employer-employee master narrative.

2. Employee health

Employee health is important for the social and economic benefits that add materially to individual and national well being. Health is bound closely, but in a complex way, to work because there is a clear relationship between income derived from work and incidence and prevalence of specific diseases and injuries (Ziglio 2000:34).

The public health policies concerning employee health are developed from collaboration between governments and business and many disciplines are involved in investigating employee health. From the *Research Fields, Courses, and Disciplines Classifications Codes* of the Australian Research Council (2004), some of the disciplines involved researching employee health and the subjects that flow from them include:

- Public health and health services
  - Health Promotion
  - Environmental and Occupational Health and Safety
- Business and Management
  - Organisational Planning and Management
- Psychology
  - Industrial and Organisational Psychology
- Engineering and Technology
  - Safety and Quality

These disciplines have different but legitimate, perspectives on employee health which influence public health policies concerning employee health and also influence the theories about occupational illness (Bohle & Quinlan 2000:66). Nevertheless, none of these individual disciplines has solved the difficulties that give rise to these policies (Quinlan 1993b:18). Taking a new approach, therefore, this research is interdisciplinary. The *immediate discipline* of this research is Health Promotion in the Workplace. Work and health, according to Schabracq, Winnubst and Cooper (1996:xiv) exist in an interdisciplinary arena, therefore the research problem is related to the parent disciplines of Public Health and Health Services, Business and Management, Psychology and Engineering and Technology. Although interdisciplinary work usually involves argument with established disciplines, this work provides productive tension to supplement and complement existing knowledge.

Over the last hundred years, theories of the causes of occupational illness have relied heavily on the evolving viewpoints of particular disciplines, for example engineering, psychology and sociology (Bohle & Quinlan 2000:66). Hale and Hovden (1998:129–131) describe a progression in the theories of occupational illness causation, extending from the early industrial period before World War I with its engineering and technical focus, through a human factors approach, to the current preoccupation with management systems. Although a comprehensive approach to employee health has developed, the complex system dynamics existing in the real workplace often mean that implementation of that approach is less than ideal (Bohle & Quinlan 2000:115–119). Hopkins (2000), in his book, *Lessons from Longford – The Esso Gas Plant Explosion* illustrates this point well. Hopkins investigates the 1999 disaster which killed two workers and cut the gas supply of the state of Victoria for two weeks. Hopkins (2000:120–124) locates the network of causes of the disaster in five levels: physical; organisational; company; government/regulation; and social, in decreasing order of proximity from the accident. In this chain of causation there was an 'absence of mindfulness' (2000:139–151) about interpreting weak signals of malfunction that existed in each of these levels. The implementation of a comprehensive approach to safety and therefore employee health is shown to be ineffective.

The two major workplace health policy responses in Australia are the Workers' Compensation system and the Occupational Health and Safety system. The Australian compensation model is workplace based and provides part of the 'the wage earner's welfare state' (Castles 1989:21). Other public and organisational policies in Australia also influence employee health, for example, Anti-discrimination and Equity legislation, Enterprise Bargaining Agreements, and Wellness programs.

Some countries have a national scheme that covers all accidents and is integrated into the social security system (Aarts & De Jong 1992; Industry Commission 1994). The performance of these approaches, whether workplace-based or integrated, is influenced more by the social control operating in institutions, organisations and groups, rather than simply in the structure of these systems (Industry Commission 1994, 1995).

The complexities and conflict that arise between multiple stakeholders with their divergent needs of workplace health policies are succinctly summarised by Johnstone (1997:544) when he wrote about Workers' Compensation policy:

> Compensation policy assumes the characteristics of a kind of morality play in a capitalist industrial society such as Australia. Interest lies not simply in the financial costs and benefits of the compensation scheme, but also in the impact of the scheme on a variety of fragile and subtle concerns such as the maintenance of work incentives, the authority of employment relations, the allocation of blame for disablement, the promotion of accident deterrence, the preservation of professional autonomy, and the acknowledgment of worker rights.

Many authors report that these workplace health policy structures fail because the benefits are too few and the costs are too high. Foley, Gale and Gavenlock (1995:171), in reviewing the costs of work-related injury and disease, found that 'there was ample scope for improvement'. Until the Kerr Report in 1996, occupationally-related mortality was seriously underreported because occupational exposures to hazardous substances and subsequent deaths were not previously regarded as work-related (Kerr et al. 1996). Pearse and Refshauge (1987:635) refer to the 'unacceptably high levels of fatalities, occupational injuries and ill health'. Mayhew and Peterson (1999b:1) support their opinion that 'prevention efforts of recent years have failed' by referring to the 2900 work-related deaths each year and the costs to Australia of work-related injury of around 5% of the Gross Domestic Product (GDP) or at least twenty billion dollars. By comparison, in 1998 there were 2030 road fatalities in Australia (WorkCover 2002a). The schemes must meet their financial obligations to supply medical treatment and lost wages to employees and are constantly under review in an attempt to fulfill these requirements. The sheer size of the financial costs involved in managing work-related injury and illness means that Workers' Compensation insurance is the second largest area of private insurance after motor vehicle insurance (Bohle & Quinlan 2000:342).

The Australian workplace has undergone changes in the last twenty years. There are increased demands from globalisation of the economy and the rapid development of communication technology. Under the pressures of economic rationalism, the workforce has been and is affected by the decentralisation of industrial relations and an almost complete reliance on enterprise bargaining for wage increases (Crittall 1995:587–593; Horstman 1999:325–341). Economic rationalism allows the free market and its competitive forces to decide economic and social priorities. Although enterprise bargaining affects critical issues like hours of work, patterns of labour, new technology, multi-skilling and piece-rate payment, Crittal's (1995:587) research found that occupational health and safety issues are largely ignored in the enterprise bargaining process. These changes have moved employee health even further from industrial negotiations (Creighton & Gunningham 1985; Quinlan 1993a:140–169).

These workplace changes have meant the decline in full-time employment and a corresponding expansion of 'precarious' employment (Quinlan & Mayhew 1999:491), that is, an increase in the use of shiftwork/nightwork, telecommuting, home-based work, part-time, multiple job holding, temporary employment and contract employment. Fragmentation of internal labour markets is an international trend according to Rubery (1999:116–137). Quinlan and Mayhew (1999:491–493) state the expansion of 'precarious' employment and the changing nature of work affect the patterns of workplace injury and disease and threaten to undermine existing regulatory regimes. As a result, workers' inputs into workplace health policy have been further reduced. Workers and their unions do not participate in the numerous inquiries into these schemes to the same degree that government officials, technical experts, lawyers and medical practitioners do (Industry Commission 1994, 1995) and at the workplace the formal requirements for employee participation through risk management 'overstate worker influence' (Per Oystein Saksvik & Quinlan 2003:37).

Although the concept of work environment was previously well-defined by its physicality (Allvin & Aronsson 2003:109), changes in work practices have expanded the concept to take account of the psychosocial environment. Problems in the psychosocial environment, for example, personnel problems, *stress, burnout,* difficulties in co-operating and harassment, involve the individual worker's ability to cope with work and his/her fellow workers. The expansion of the concept is associated increased recognition that the workplaces are politicised and there is increased complexity regarding employers' responsibilities (Allvin & Aronsson 2003:99–111).

There are changing views about health in contemporary society (Grbich 1996, George & Davis 1998) and these views do not rely only on the biomedical model of orthodox Western medicine in which health is viewed as the individual's responsibility; is defined as the absence of illness (Holmes, Hughes & Julian 2003:250); and is driven by the interests of corporations (Lax 2002:519). The main challenge to the biomedical view of health is its ineffectiveness in the context of escalating costs of health care (Nettleton 1995:5-8). Changing views of health incorporate the following: the consumers' perspective of health; epidemiological studies of health inequalities that show the rich enjoy better health than the poor (Holmes, Hughes & Julian 2003:278); and sociological studies about health and illness as socially constructed phenomena (Dembe 1996, 1999; Illich 1977; Marmot 1996; Navarro 1978). This has contributed to a broader and more ecological view of health than the biomedical model alone envisions (Murray 2001:220).

A multi-dimensional view of health is now considered to have social, mental, spiritual, emotional and physical elements (Cribbs & Dines 1993). This view of health is reflected in documents like the Ottawa Charter for Health Promotion (WHO 1986). Health promotion according to the Charter is:

> the process of enabling people to increase control over, and improve their health. To reach a state of complete physical, mental and social well being, an individual or group must be able to identify and realise aspirations, to satisfy needs and to change or cope with the environment. Health is, therefore, seen as a resource for everyday life, not the objective of living. Health is a positive concept emphasising social and personal resources, as well as physical capacities.

The Charter also recognises that the organisation of work should help create a healthy society. In creating supportive environments at work, workplace health promotion changes from a singular focus on individual behaviour to 'recognition of the broader social, environmental and economic determinants of health' (O'Connor-Fleming & Parker 2001:231).

The multi-dimensional view of health has not yet penetrated far into the regulatory regimes that influence employee health. In Australia, as in the United Kingdom, there is an historical and legislative separation of health services and prevention strategies in the general community as well as for employees. Wilkinson (2001:152) describes this process in the workplace with health promotion and occupational health and safety operating in isolation from each other and having different intervention targets, personnel and methods.

There has been a clear line of development with the notion of workplace impacting on health since the WHO strategy of *Health for All* in 1980 and the 1986 Ottawa Charter for Health Promotion. Subsequent milestone health promotion documents, for example, Sundsvall Statement 1992, Jakarta Declaration 1997 ratified and refined the idea of 'settings' for health. A setting is a 'place or social context in which people engage in daily activities in which environmental, organizational, and personal factors interact to affect health and wellbeing' (Health Promotion Glossary, 1988). However, the workplace as a setting for health campaigns infringes on the free enterprise philosophy of neoliberalism, marketplace practices, and the business owners' prerogatives. Business and governments control workplace policy with employees being subordinate to other stakeholders. This is a problem and I will discuss why it is a problem now. The 'settings' approach in the Ottawa Charter recognises that the social, psychological and physical contexts in which people live and work shape their opportunities and choices in relation to health. This approach has been applied to employee health in a variety of workplaces settings including universities (Dooris 2001:58).

Current workplace health policies develop out of a certain political economy. Considine (1991:7) defines this political economy as the landscape in which the principal actors move. This landscape is made up of policy environment that deals with economic and organisational relationships and government authority. Throughout the history of Workers Compensation and Occupational Health and Safety legislation there has been resistance to workers' claims and opinions. This echoes the adversarial approach to all other employer/employees affairs. This present research addresses an imbalance that has existed in who determines the shape of those policies. Giddens (1979:5) makes the point that people can influence the social structures in which they live.

3. Employment and ill health is a neglected reality

3.1 Legislation is not entirely adequate

Much of the more recent health promotion literature and public health literature has an awareness of collective rather than just individual responsibility for health, hence the notion in the Ottawa Charter of 'strengthening supportive environments'. Although it can be argued that there is legislation to protect employees, its collective contribution to individual health is not entirely adequate. For example, the pragmatic political process involving governments, business and professions ensures that workplace health policy is subjected to myths of crisis over compensation funding obligations, but in essence, harm to workers may not be reduced (Mayhew & Peterson, 1999a:2). The ability of individual workers to look after their health is compromised by their lack of power in a system that does not optimise the potential synergies between individual and collective action. Workplace governance prioritises organisational production over employee welfare and the workers do not have power and/or knowledge to control risks in the work environment (Ziglio, 1991:69).

3.2 Complex organisational experiences and dimensions of health and ill health

When taking a limited individualist's approach to health it follows that if the workplace is unsatisfactory them the employee should leave. In reality work is not that simple. Some workers respond to negative organisational experiences by leaving, but according to Australian workforce statistics (ABS, 2000:1) about stability of workers, they are more likely to stay at work and respond with poor service, difficult working relationships, poor quality work, lack of innovation, poor decision making, and low productivity. Williams and Cooper (1999:9) refer to this sub optimal performance as the 'hidden health issue' for organisations, whereas, sickness absence and staff turnover are the 'visible' and more obvious signs of poor health and well being. These two factors, that is, the performance of workers, and the stability of the workforce, mean that the workers' responses to organisational experiences may be complex and attenuated, and impact on the organisation's functioning in diverse ways.

Terkel's view of work (1972:xi) captures the chronic nature of the work situation that is in stark contrast to the simplistic assumptions that suggest that a worker can move to another job if s/he is not happy at work:

> Work by its very nature is about violence to the spirit as well as the body. It is about ulcers as well as accidents, about shouting matches as well as fist fights, about nervous breakdowns as well as kicking the dog around. It is above all (or beneath all), about daily humiliations. To survive the day is triumph for the walking wounded among the great many of us.

Terkel's words bring home the chronicity of workplace stress, rather than the novelty and intensity of acute stress that disrupts goal directed behaviour and is of relatively short duration. Sometimes, no single source of chronic stress may seem to be of consequence but the combined or cumulative effects of these stressors can lead to poor performance over time, reduced well being, health problems and decreased ability to respond effectively to acute stress demands (Driskell & Salas, 1996:7).

The complex nature of workers' responses to organisational experiences and the dimensions of health and ill health over the usual forty-year period of the lifespan in employment are very important to employees and employers. The health effects and the productivity effects involved provide strong justification for researching this area.

3.3 The health of workers is a measure of how the benefits of society are shared

The consequences of workplace health policies challenge the moral stance in the market justice/social justice divide. It argues for the utilitarian view, as opposed to the Rawlsian view (Rawls 1978; Weimer & Vining, 1999:135–137). The utilitarian view is one approach to public policy in which the expected outcomes are distributed in democratic and egalitarian ways to all participants. The Rawlsian view on the other hand would distribute the greatest benefits to the least advantaged in the community. The utilitarian view of public policy does not guarantee minimal allocation to individuals and the Rawlsian view does not provide incentives for those who create wealth.

Governments must walk the line between developing and implementing policies that provide incentives to business yet at the same time meet the needs of their least advantaged and least powerful constituents, the workers. This work will document the opinions of workers and therefore assist governments in their decision making about the distributional rationale.

3.4 Sometimes experts' opinions do not acknowledge social reality

Although the state, employers, unions the professions and experts design and implement policy and structures for employees' wellbeing workplace health policies are not a contained and successful program. Unfortunately, the numbers of deaths that occur in Australian workplaces indicate a different reality (Mayhew & Peterson, 1999:6). In the manner of Wildavsky (1979:3), who suggests speaking out clearly about social problems, this work aims to seek workers' 'truths' and to deliver the findings about those truths in a way that will influence the political economy of policies that bear on employee health.

It is the nature of truth, according to Lupton (1995:160–161), to be 'transitory and political, and the position of subjects to be inevitably fragmentary and contradictory' however, workers' truth is 'one of the varieties of truth' enmeshed in discursive practices of the workplace. Therefore, when this truth is presented it may redress the imbalance that currently exists in the conventional perspectives of employee health.

4. Employment and the burden of illness

Much of the literature on occupational health and safety has a technical edge that addresses the physical aspects of risks and the physical aspects of injury. Nevertheless, the rate of injury is impressive. Statistical data is used extensively by government authorities, like WorkCover (1997–1998), to provide a basis for the 'national scorecard' in managing employee health. Aggregate data do not give an adequate portrayal of any social problem when considered by themselves, because the reader is not drawn into the human story embedded within the quantitative data. Not only is the personal side of the scorecard lost, there are shortcomings in statistic data itself. Mandryk et al. (2001:359) point out that the data often underestimates the problem, and there is a lack of information on causes of injuries and a lack of information on the relationship between injuries and outcomes for the injured worker.

Nevertheless, the following statistics that deal with injuries and illnesses in the Australian workforce have been compiled from a number of authors who comment on the extent of workplace injury and disease. The sources for this data are: Industry Commission 1995:Vol 1, Pxix, Vol 11, P19–33; Driscoll & Mayhew 1999:28–51; Driscoll et al. 2001:45–66; Ellis 2001:xxiv-xxv; Emmett 1999; Foley, Gale & Gavenlock 1995; Foley 1997; Johnstone 1997:13–14; Kerr et al. 1996; Mandryk et al. 2001: 349–361; Mayhew & Peterson 1999b:1–13; Stiller, Sargaison & Mitchell 1998:25.

Mortality:
- there are 2900 deaths each year as a result of work-related injury and illness —
  a significant number of these deaths are due to occupational cancers from exposure to hazardous material (Mayhew & Peterson 1999:6)
- there are 603 work-related traumatic deaths per year (Driscoll et al. 2001:45).

Injury:
- up to 650,000 workers, that is, one in twelve workers, suffer injury or illness from work
- there is a trend towards an increase of serious injuries causing permanent disability (Stiller, Sargaison & Mitchell 1998:25)

Occupational disease:
- the incidence of occupational disease is likely to rise related to the recognition of several factors:
  - chronicity (which refers to the long length of exposure, e.g. noise-induced hearing loss and musculo-skeletal disorders)
  - latency (which refers to the length of time from exposure to appearance of the disease e.g. asbestosis occurs about twenty years after exposure)
  - the multifactorial nature of illness (Ellis 2001:xxiv-xxv)

- the significant underestimation of the level of occupational injury and disease is addressed (Bohle & Quinlan 2000:35–40)
- work-related health problems affect people after retirement
  - up to 300,000 persons over the age of sixty-five are estimated to be suffering from work-related health problems

Costs:

- direct Workers' Compensation costs constitute 1.5% of GNP or 5% of GDP, at least twenty billion dollars (Industry Commission 1995:99)
- workers compensation costs are 20% of total health care costs
- of the total costs of workplace injury and disease:
  - 30% are borne by the injured worker and their families
  - 40% are borne by the employers in lost productivity
  - 30% are borne by the community in social security payments and health subsidies (Industry Commission 1995:102)

Equity:

- Workers' Compensation figures seriously understate the extent of occupational disease (Foley, Gale & Gavenlock 1995:171)
- some groups, (for example, the self-employed), are not entitled to make Workers' Compensation claims for work-related injury and disease
- some groups are reluctant to make claims, particularly workers from non-English speaking backgrounds, and those in precarious employment (Bohle & Quinlan 2000:35–46).

Dr. Yossi Berger (1999:52), Head of the Occupational Health and Safety unit of the Australian Workers Union, states that what matters at work is the workers 'expressed views about occupational reality'. He describes these expressed views as the 'mumbling environment' to emphasise that workers are living and experiencing this harm at work but no one is listening to them.

In the same vein, Wilkinson expands this view of the social reality of employee health when she speaks about employee sickness not being related just to technical exposures of harmful agents, but more related to how people treat each other in the work environment. She states that: '[Employee injury or ill health] is not simply a biological process triggered by chemicals, or the fabric of the organisation. It is stimulated and perpetuated by its people through group processes, action and behaviour at every level of the organisation' (Wilkinson 2001:24).

Bohle and Quinlan (1991:92) emphasise that harm to employees is usually not sudden and unexpected. On the contrary, there is a definite probability of harm. The reality for workers is that there is a probability of work-related injury and illness because the patterns of injuries between occupational and industry groups are consistent over time. In 2000, Bohle and Quinlan (2000:46) said that 'work-related injuries and illnesses constitute statistical probabilities' and this undermines any attempt to portray them and illnesses as 'unexpected or aberrant events'. The familiarity of workers with injury and work-related disease has contributed to their 'deep-seated cynicism and skepticism' at work about the workplace being safe for them (Berger 1999:58).

4.1 Employment and the burden of mental illness

The Employment Conditions Knowledge Network (EMCONET) delivered its final report to the Commission of Social Determinants of Health in 2007 on the neglected global reality of employment conditions and health inequalities. The Report takes the view that health inequalities derive from social injustice that has its origins in the distribution of resources in society that, in turn is determined by political decisions. From an historical point of view the Medical professions link to business and free enterprise has been slow to relate specific work conditions to occupational illness and generally policy development is dominated by the interests of business and governments with the contribution of employees being subordinate to these other stakeholders (Per Oystein Saksvik & Quinlan 2003:37).

Employment relations refer to the relationship between the employer and the worker who is hired to sell or produce goods through his labour and he is paid wages. Employment relations in the formal economy of developed nations may be contractual, but in the informal economy of many developing countries employment relations are personal agreements in which the power differential between employer and employee has not protection under law or by employee unionisation. Employment conditions refer to the types of employment arrangements that exist between employer and employee. Some are, unemployment, precarious employment, informal employment and informal jobs, child labour, and slavery/bonded labour. Working conditions deal with the tasks performed by workers, the way work is organised, the physical and chemical work environment, ergonomics, the psychosocial work environment, and the technology used.

Table 1. Definitions of three interrelated concepts

This Report takes a broader view beyond individual hazards involved in working conditions to consider the 'political, cultural and economic context to provide a comprehensive account of the current international situation of labour markets and types of employment conditions' (EMCONET, 2007 p. 14).

The three interconnected concepts of employment relations, employment conditions and work conditions are taken together in this report because the first two concepts are key social determinants in shaping health inequalities. The three provide a much better understanding of burden of illness that employment causes due to inequalities.

Fair employment is a concept that incorporates factors of employment relations, employment conditions and working conditions that promote workers' good health and well being. These factors would be:

- Freedom from coercion
- Job security
- Fair income
- Job protection that includes social security
- Respect and dignity at work
- Workplace participation
- Enrichment and lack of alienation

The Report's macro-theoretical framework of employment relations and health inequalities relies heavily on the framework for explaining social and economic disease patterns developed by Dahlgren and Whitehead in 1991 and reproduced by Marmot (1996:66). This framework emphasises the primacy of age, sex and hereditary factors. The clinical approach to disease focuses on these factors and individual behaviour. Research into prevention has generally been concerned with individual risk factors for disease, for example smoking and drinking. Living and working, social and community influences, and general socio-economic, cultural and environmental conditions have attracted less research. Figure 1 shows the relationships that exist through power differentials in employment relations, through labour market and social welfare policies that are played out in employment conditions and work conditions causing health inequalities.

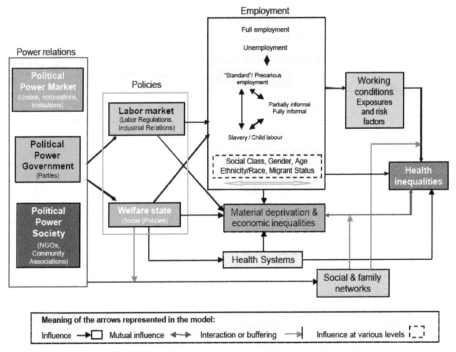

Fig. 1. Macro-theoretical framework of employment relations and health inequalities
Source: EMCONET (2007, p. 31).

This macro-theoretical framework shows the interconnected nature of the political processes that influence employee health.

At the micro-theoretical level the Report provides a framework of employment conditions and health inequalities. At this micro level the resulting working conditions shape health behaviours, provoke physio-pathological changes and determine psychsocial factors that influence mental wellbeing.

The effects of many of these factors in Figure 1 and 2 and compounded in real world situation. For example material deprivation and economic inequalities is characterised by poor nutrition, poverty, poor housing and low income, and they develop from lack of welfare policies in many developing countries and employment conditions where there is little social justice, for example those in the informal economy. Material deprivation and economic inequalities have an 'effect on chronic diseases and mental health via severe psychological factors life-style behaviours ad physio-pathological changes' EMCONET 2007, p. 33).

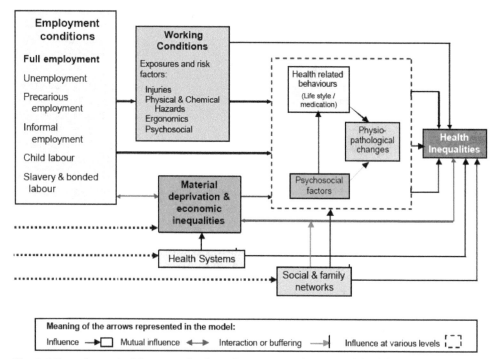

Fig. 2. Micro-theoretical framework of employment conditions and health inequalities
Source: EMCONET (2007, p. 32).

There is much in the literature on psychosocial theories about the importance of social stratification or where one stands in relation to others, and its effect on health and mental wellbeing. Marmot (1996:63) uses Dahlgren and Whitehead's framework to describe his significant findings about the social patterns of disease. Marmot and a group of researchers known as the Whitehall team have advanced understanding in this area, particularly in relation to the patterning of disease in the social hierarchy at work. The Whitehall research involves a longitudinal study of 10,308 male and female British civil servants and was started in 1985. Marmot and Theorell (1988:659–673) report there is a steep inverse association between grade of employment and mortality from coronary heart disease and a range of other causes. In Whitehall II, Stansfield, Head and Marmot (2000) use the General Health Questionnaire and the SF-36, as well as other measures, and sickness absence of both short spells (1–7 days) and long spells (8 days or more). Stansfield, Head and Marmot's findings show that low decision latitude, high job demands, low social support, and the combination of high effort and low rewards are associated with poor mental health and poor health functioning. Their results suggest that intervention at the level of work design, organisation and management might reduce morbidity in working populations.

Marmot's work in the Whitehall I and Whitehall II studies show a social gradient in mortality and morbidity. Morbidity and mortality rates are higher for those at the bottom of the social hierarchy than at the top. Van Rossum et al. (2000:178) also report from the Whitehall II study to show that the mortality differentials persist at older ages for almost all causes of death in this 'white collar' cohort. The mortality rates are higher in the lowest grades of employment. More specifically, the workers at each point in the hierarchy have worse health than those above them and better health than those of lower rank. In effect, this indicates that social, cultural, working and economic factors, have a strong influence on biology. This work emphasises the social and biological pathways that underlie the social patterning of disease (Marmot 1996, 1998:403; Marmot Shipley & Rose 1984).

In the United Kingdom, the Acheson Report (1998:33) into Inequalities in Health is adamant that policy emphasis should be made 'upstream' from the individual (i.e. targeting the factors in the outer boxes of the Dahlgren and Whitehead framework) to the social and economic structures if any worthwhile changes in health inequalities are to be made, because comparatively little is accomplished by addressing 'downstream' influences of individual lifestyle, age, sex, and hereditary factors (i.e. the inner boxes of the framework).

Results from the Australian Health Promotion Survey of 1994 reported by Harris Sainsbury and Nutbeam (1999) support the differentials in health status and exposure to risk that are found in the Whitehall studies. Lower education levels, unemployment rather than employment status, areas of residence of socio-economic disadvantage, living alone, and rural compared to urban residence are associated with poorer health status. On the other hand belonging to a particular immigrant group was not associated with a difference of health status (Harris Sainsbury & Nutbeam 1999:19–31). These researchers find that structural factors, that is, poor quality of social and economic environments account for most of the health status differentials observed. In Australia it is a problem of relative disadvantage rather than absolute lack of resources for these groups that experience health inequities. This type of research is the background for Petersen and Lupton's (1996) opinions about the diverse causal pathways that influence disease patterns in society rather than the simplistic interpretation of Dahlgren and Whitehead's framework that implies genetics, age and sex are the sole or primary determinants of health status.

In the literature on work and health three theories are so frequently mentioned that they are referred to here:
- Demand-Control-Support (Karasek 1979)
- Person–Environment Fit (Caplan 1983)
- Effort-Reward (Siegrist 1998:190–204, Siegrist & Theorell 2006).

Wilkinson's list of social determinants of health in the workplace include:
- Demand-control (Karasek 1979)1
- Support with work processes (Cohen & Syme 1985; Winnubst & Schabracq 1996:87–104)
- Stimulation (Edwards, Caplan & Van Harrison 1998:28–67)
- Effort –reward (Siegrist's 1998:190-204)
- Ability to unwind (Gutek, Repetti & Silver 1988:141-174).
- Participation (Holbeche 1998:30–35)

Table 2. Psychosocial theories of work and health

These three theories help to explain the action of the psychosocial factors that affect the individual worker's health in the work environment. Briefly, the Demand-Control-Support theory relates the demands placed on workers with the degree of control that they have over those demands and the support that they perceive is offered to them in doing the work. The Person-Environment Fit describes the satisfaction that is derived from the worker being appropriately skilled and adjusted to the work situation. The Effort-Reward theory links the inducements or rewards that the organisation offers to the effort that the worker has to put into work.

Wilkinson (2001) in the preface to her book, Fundamentals of Health at Work refers to the 'neglected social context of workplaces', and within the text provides a list of the social determinants of health in the workplace and the theories behind some of those concepts (2001:9–10). The sources of these social determinants vary in the work environment. Some relate to the job itself, to the worker's role in the organisation, to the worker's aspirations and career development, to relationships at work, and/or to the organisational structure or culture of the workplace (Sutherland & Cooper 1988:3–31). A modified form of Wilkinson's list includes the following concepts:

- Demand-Control: The Demand-Control-Support model was first developed by Karasek. (Karasek 1979; Karasek & Theorell 1990; Theorell 1998). Demand incorporates the concept of quantitative work overload or underload, that is, too many or too few tasks, whereas qualitative work overload or underload refers to tasks that the worker does not feel capable of doing. In essence, constraints on decision making or decision latitude, rather than decision making itself are a major problem. Decision latitude or control, or the degree of autonomy that a worker has in performing work tasks, is a central component of this model and has been found to be closely related to job satisfaction. This affects not only executives but also workers in lower status jobs with little freedom to make decisions. The most adverse reactions of physical strain, anxiety and depression can occur when the psychological demands of the job are high and the workers decisions latitude in the task is low (Karasek 1989; Karasek & Theorell 1990). Lack of control over working systems has been found to lead to stress and predisposes to cardio-vascular disease (Marmot et al. 1998). The ability to plan work tasks involves several aspects of control in the work environment. Role conflict, ambiguity, overplanning and work methods, all of which mean that the employee has a lack of control, predispose the individual to stress (Sutherland & Cooper 1988:3–31). Role conflict occurs when compliance with one set of role pressures makes compliance with another set of role pressures impossible. Role ambiguity refers to inadequate or misleading information about how a person is supposed to do the job (Ross & Altmanier 1994).

- Support with work processes: The support component of Karasek's model of Demand–Control–Support refers to optimal matching of the amount and type of support appropriate to a work situation with its particular demands, and the amount of decision latitude available to the worker in that situation. There are different types of supports provided in the workplace through relationships with peers and supervisors. These human ties are important in mental and physical health (Cohen & Syme 1985; Winnubst & Schabracq 1996:87–104).

- Stimulation: De-skilling and fragmentation of tasks has been linked to stress. The person must 'fit' into the work environment (Edwards, Caplan & Van Harrison 1998:28–67). This fit in the Person–Environment Fit model refers to the match between what the worker expects and what the job actually requires. As well as expectations, the skill of the worker fuses with what the job requires (Cox 1978). The person-in-environment psychology has been extended by Wapner and Demick (2000:27) to be holistic, developmental and systems orientated.

- Effort–Reward: Siegrist's Effort–Reward model (1998:190-204) proposes that there is an appropriate balance between the rewards that the worker expects and the efforts needed to obtain those rewards. Workers act formally and informally to change their work environment so that inequities between what they offer and what they get, and what they perceive other workers receive in relation to what they contribute, are removed. Using different terminology but dealing with similar concepts as the Person–Environment fit and Effort–Reward, Williams (1993) refers to the congruent person and organisation. Congruency is achieved by merging belief systems, values, plans and strategies so 'so that we can gracefully move through life being congruent and functional' (1993:165). Although Williams is casting his argument in terms of the ideal, there is no doubt some validity in the optimisation of enhancing employee personal strength and enhancing the creative potential of the organisation.
- Ability to unwind: To recover vitality through interpersonal relationships at work and through relationships and interests in the home domain is necessary because of the persistent requirements of work. The circular and reciprocal relationships between work and non-work or work and home domain are important because the balance in these linkages affects quality of life for the worker and his/her significant others (Gutek, Repetti & Silver 1988:141-174).
- Participation: Participation of employees in the work effort varies from optimal performance producing maximum productivity, to hostility that sabotages productivity. Holbeche (1998:30-35) found the more common response from employees experiencing poor work conditions was non-participation which meant holding back on human resources. The most extreme problem of this kind is called 'presenteeism', which occurs when employees come to work but contribute little to the work effort because they are distressed by their jobs or some aspect of the work environment (Schabracq, Winnubst & Cooper 2003:xv). Aronsson, Gustafsson and Dallner's study (2000:502) into 'sickness presenteeism' shows that members of occupational groups whose everyday tasks are to provide care, welfare services, teach or instruct have an increased risk of being at work when sick, which is itself a form of presenteeism.
- Emotional work: Performance of emotional work in the long-term, particularly in the caring professions and service industries, like teaching, can produce a 'burnout syndrome' that is characterised by mental exhaustion, cynicism and loss of commitment (Maslach 1982, 1998:68-85; Maslach & Jackson 1986:253-266).

5. Contemporary employment issues in developed and developing countries

The culture of a group is very influential for health. Culture is defined as:
a complex integrated system that includes knowledge, beliefs, skills, art, morals, law, customs, and other acquired habits and capabilities of the human being. (Murray, Zentner & Samiezade-Yard 2001:4).
A culture is both ideal, in that it aspires to certain values and health beliefs, and it is also manifest. The manifest culture is the expression of the way people think and behave. Within the dominant culture there are subcultures — groups of people within a larger culture, of the same age, socioeconomic level, occupation, or with the same goals, who have an identity of their own but are related to the total culture in certain ways. For example, regional culture refers to the local or regional manifestations of a larger culture (Murray & Zentner, 2001:5). In the same way, workgroups and organisations form subcultures of the larger societal

culture. Workgroups share industry and professional allegiances, and organisations develop cultures related to their founder, origins and evolutionary experiences. The health status of a workgroup derives much from the organisational culture and wider community culture to which the workers and organisation belong.

Cultures, however, are not static entities. They are subject to changes. For example, in Western modern society some of the cultural problem areas and trends that Murray, Zentner and Samiezade-Yard (2001:9) note include:

- need for more professional knowledge
- greater expectation of the public for services and quality of services
- more goods considered to be public goods
- lack of measurement to show what is actually needed, and thus where the money and resources should be directed
- short-term rather than long-term considerations in the business economy, health services and social service
- changing demography and more urban concentration
- increased life expectancy
- changing values with little understanding of the historical roots of the culture
- power struggles between groups.

From this list two unifying themes in contemporary cultural changes are individualism and economic rationalism and it is necessary to understand their impact on health and work (Murray, Zentner and Samiezade-Yard 2001:9). These themes are significant in the tertiary education industry because of their effect on the nature of educational services offered and the means of delivery of those services. Technology also shapes the educational workplace and other service industries through its impact services and service delivery.

5.1 Individualism

According to Naisbitt and Aburdene (1990:299) the doctrine of individual responsibility was a major cultural trend in the last decades of the 20th century. Individualism fosters a climate of 'independence', with freely choosing individuals who do not need to care about others individually or collectively. Notwithstanding the self reliance that individualism ostensibly creates, Naisbitt and Aburdene acknowledge that society as a whole gains by the action of individuals when they achieve in any area of human endeavour.

Cultures also vary in the degree to which they balance the interplay of collectivism and individualism. Strongly collective cultures are tightly bound and cohesive and expect unswerving loyalty, whereas individual cultures are those in which connections between people are loose and individuals are expected to look after themselves. Cultures that are collectively bound usually have power distance dimensions within them. Power distance is defined as 'the extent to which less powerful members of organisations expect and accept that power is distributed unequally' (Erez & Earley 1993:104). Culture influences both systems and individual behaviour and is influenced by them (Anthony 1994:2). The tension between individualism and collectivism, which is a cultural characteristic of the wider society and organisations and workplaces, is translated in the workplace through the concepts of personal social capital, social capital and community capacity. The development of organisations and workplaces and the health of individuals at work are interactional and the level of trust between employees, who are usually not related by family ties, impacts on their health.

5.2 Personal social capital, social capital and community capacity

At the personal level, social capital refers to strength of personal support networks and ability to access such support, as well as trust, mutual responsibility and effective collaboration (Putnam 2000:19–26). Social capital also operates at the level of society, in a set of complex interactions between community level characteristics, such as trust, participation and cooperation evident in values, norms and connections that allow people to work together for the common good. Trust operates at the micro level of the interaction between people and is regarded as the 'most valuable factor' in social capital (Berry & Rickwood 2000:36). Trust is most valuable to the social capital of an organisation because it allows people to support each other. Through trust employees are free to be open and to achieve their potential in life (Bruhn 2001:38).

Putnam (2000:19) clarified the differences between physical capital, human capital and social capital thus: physical capital refers to physical objects; human capital refers to properties of individuals; and social capital refers to connections among individuals, social networks and norms of reciprocity and trustworthiness that arise from them. This is not a romantic view of social capital (Baum 1999:195) or a costless way of making society and the economy work better (Wilkinson 2000:411), or a preference for psychosocial conditions over material conditions (Lynch et al. 2000:404). Navarro (2002:427) does not accept the use of the term 'social capital' because, he states, Putnam does not consider power and politics as factors that affect an individual's ability to compete for resources but considers only participation and togetherness. A more balanced view however, sees social capital as strongly influenced by political, legal and corporate action rather than simply being individually determined (Lynch et al. 2002:407). Social capital can be fostered or not through the way social networks and supports are developed and encouraged by governments and organisations. Collective action to increase social capital can be a public strategy to overcome some socio-economic inequalities and improve health.

Social capital operates at two levels—bonds and bridges. Bonds refer to the strength of internal relationships in the group and bridges refer to the capacity of the group to connect to other societies (Kreuter & Lezin 2002: 239), whereas the concept 'community capacity' relates to the ability of the community to change constructively in relation to social and public health problems (Norton et al. 2002:194–227).

The dimension of individualism—collectivism existing in a particular workplace—is demonstrated by the social capital and community capacity that work teams and the organisation have at their disposal to cope with change. The social relationships involved determine health status and productivity. Therefore, the dimension of individualism—collectivism and the corresponding social capital and community capacity—are the group level constructs that operate in the work subculture and influence employee health.

5.3 Economic rationalism

A second unifying theme in the cultural changes effecting post-industrial society is economic rationalism. Economic rationalism is a form of ideological reasoning which took hold in the 1980s in Australia and is based on the notion that the free market is a much better arbiter of economic and other matters than are governments (Pusey 1991). Economic rationalism sees itself as a science largely devoid of social goals, and the language and logic of economics begins to dominate social policy. A corollary of such reasoning is a reduction in spending by the state on such things as education, health and social welfare, and a shift in providing these services to the private sector (Holmes, Hughes & Julian 2003:231).

Economic rationalism and capitalism sit more easily with profit making businesses. However, the provision of public goods by public institutions such as hospitals, universities and schools, is achieved nowadays by producing these public goods in a cost-conscious competitive environment with the same awareness of the 'tyranny of the bottom line' that profit driven organisations experience (Estes 1996).

The interplay between culture and economic theory has had an illustrious recorded history in the work of classical sociologists, as for example, in Marx's *The Economic and Philosophic Manuscripts of 1844* (Marx 1964; Tucker 1978) and continues in the work of Braverman (1974). In his book, *Economic Rationalism in Canberra*, Pusey (1991:10) points out that the priorities of economic rationalism are the economy, political order and then social order. Opposition to economic rationalism is seen as cultural resistance to a 'necessary condition' or as 'rancour against (post) modernity' (1991:21).

The challenge for the 21st century is the impact of these cultural trends and their underlying themes of individualism and economic rationalism on social capital. Economic life is pervaded by culture and depends on the moral bonds of trust (Bruhn 2001:5). In the business world trust is the unspoken, unwritten bond that is a prerequisite for the legal bond because it facilitates transactions.

5.4 Technology

Technology is part of modern life and shapes many cultural dimensions and operates as part of the socio-economic, cultural and environmental conditions (i.e. included within the outer layer of Dahlgren and Whitehead's framework of patterns of disease). Cairncross (2001) predicts a business and lifestyle revolution based on technological supremacy. In his book, *The Death of Distance* (2001), Cairncross discusses cultures and communication networks that will hold businesses together through technology rather than rigid management structures. Additionally, he believes the line between home and work will blur, with more work being performed at home. The social consequences of these changes and their impact on the health of employees have not been fully researched, according to Konradt, Schmook and Malecke (2000:90).

The view of culture as resistant and therefore 'bad' occurs frequently in writings on policy implementation at the national and organisational level of strategy development and implementation (Mintzberg & Quinn 1998). Nevertheless, culture is essentially the binding force that regiments those within the culture through its cohesive action. It defends the insiders by placing boundaries around them that distinguishes them from outsiders. Thus, rather than being resistant, culture is, according to Erez and Earley (1993:104), the moderator of change.

5.5 Socio-economic status

Several authors in Australia mention that social class not only determines values, attitudes and lifestyle, but also determines health (Bates & Linder-Pelz 1987:20-25; Harris, Sainsbury & Nutbeam 1999:16-35; Lupton & Najman 1995; Palmer & Short 1994:243; Russell & Schofield 1986:51-65; Short 1999: 90-95; Turrell 1995:113-135). For example, people with higher socio-economic levels, (i.e. those with good income, higher education, and full employment) experience better health and have medical insurance, use private medical facilities and often live longer. Graycar and Jamrozik, in their review of Australia's social policy, find that as far as employment benefits are concerned, men, higher income earners and executives, administrators, professionals and sales personnel have considerable advantages over women, low income earners and lower grade occupations (1993:201). Using education as a marker for socio-economic status, Steenland, Henley and Thun (2002:11) report that life expectancy is shorter for the least versus the most educated in their 37-year follow up study of two million people in the American Cancer Society Cohort. Harris, Sainsbury and Nutbeam (1999:43) state that:

> It is generally accepted that the most powerful influence on differences in health across population groups is relative poverty and associated structural forces, which serve to increase and maintain the differences. One's position in society's economic hierarchy determines choices of health promoting activity directly through access to resources such as goods and services, and indirectly through social expectations and opportunities.

Those people who belong to lower socio-economic groups lack power in social and political relationships, and may be vulnerable to workplace bullying. Research on workplace bullying identify employees whose health is affected by that experience. The victims of bullying are often subordinated or discriminated against, marginalised or disenfranchised, and suffer mental health problems as a result of the bullying (Hoel, Rayner & Cooper 1999:195–231). Victims of bullying experience more illness and a lower quality of life overall, and there are more premature deaths among the group members than comparable groups. Individuals in the middle and upper socio-economic levels who lack power in workplace structures may also be vulnerable to workplace bullying.

5.6 Risk

Risk is a social construct that assumes great importance in health and work literature as a means of quantifying a potential health problem. Risk is defined as:

> the exposure to possible loss, injury or danger; the probability of occurrence of a particular event (Murray, Zentner & Samiezade-Yard 2001:53)

> a probability of an adverse outcome, or a factor that raises this probability (World Health Organization 2002:1).

Risk factors are characteristics associated with an increased probability of a particular event, usually an injury or illness occurring (Murray, Zentner & Samiezade-Yard 2001:53). Risk assessment is part of the process of weighing up health problems and trying to be effective and efficient with interventions to benefit the individual and community. The regulation of risk involves attempts to control risk by setting and enforcing behavioural and product standards.

Within the workplace in Australia, the assessment and control of health risks is the responsibility of management through Occupational Health and Safety legislation, but this self regulation is far from effective. In an effort to improve this, the Australian government has appointed Richard Johnstone and Neil Gunningham to the National Research Centre for OHS Regulation to initiate, encourage and support research into OHS regulation (Johnstone 2002:4).

According to the Australian Bureau of Statistics report on the *Social Trends for Health: Risk Factors among Adults* (2003), the risk factor responsible for the greatest disease burden in Australia is tobacco smoking. Another common risk is excessive alcohol consumption. Excess alcohol consumption is linked to some cancers, liver disease, pancreatitis, diabetes and epilepsy. Smoking and drinking together account for about 17% of all disease

(Australian Institute Health Welfare 2000:146–148). The risk factors of smoking and excessive alcohol intake have been studied extensively.

Beck's *Risk Society* (1992) offers fair warning about the deceptive simplicity of the concept of risk in modern society. According to Beck (1992:3) risk is an 'intellectual and political web' cast by modern industrial society, in terms of problems (or risks) for the individual. These risks for the individual are conveyed in scientific language that ignores social rationality. Risks seem to concentrate in society at the lower end of the socio-economic spectrum. For example, lower socio-economic groups or those who are less powerful consume more tobacco. Also in the workplace, the least well paid workers not only operate in more hazardous environments, their amenities (e.g. tea rooms, wash rooms, etc.) are usually more limited than workers who attract higher wages. Their opportunities to have a break from work and refresh themselves, as well as their opportunities to move to better work environments are also constrained. Beck (1992:35) makes the point that 'risks seem to strengthen, not abolish the class system', on the other hand [the] 'wealthy [i.e. those with high incomes, power and education] could purchase safety and freedom from risk'.

Lupton (1995:77–105), Nettleson (1996:37, 53) and Petersen and Lupton (1996:18–20) comment on the pervasiveness of risk in literature of health and lifestyles and the limited ability that people have to control the social circumstances of their lives. These authors agree with Beck that more advantaged people have more control over socio-economic, environmental, living and working conditions. Therefore concentrating on lifestyle factors only, rather than cultural and socio-economic factors, may contribute to increasing health inequalities because advantaged people will gain doubly—from their own power base to control external factors influencing their health, and societies renewed push to enhance better lifestyle choices.

5.7 Developing countries

Notwithstanding some relatively small dips, Western economies have achieved great prosperity since Industrialisation. However the developing countries have not been so fortunate. One of the difficulties has been the lack of rule of law upon which trade relies, and the lack of modernisation. It is wrong to say that there is global integration of trade but there is some regional integration. The high-income economies represent 11.5 per cent of the world's population and produces 74 per cent of total GDP, whereas East Asia and the Pacific produce less that 7 percent, and Latin America and the Caribbean only produce 5.4 per cent (EMCONET 2007, p. 35). This inequality means that workers in developing countries are generally poorer than they compatriots in developed countries.

In developing countries there are usually less social protection standards, and employment relations and employment conditions are informal and workers are not protected by International Labour Organisation standards (ILO) and unionisation. Although the agricultural sector is still important to many developing countries it is usually done in a low productivity manner. It is mainly a family concern producing enough for the annual needs of the family and very little extra if any, compared to high productivity and high technologically driven broad area productivity in the agricultural industry in North America. There is significant rural-urban migration in some developing countries as the young and the healthy go to urban areas to seek a better life. Rural depopulation occurs when numbers of working age people migrate from the countryside to earn more money in the city. They leave behind the old and the young. For the Less Economically Developed

Countries (LEDC) the problems that develop with the influx of these rural migrants into urban areas are shanty housing, lack of clean water, pollution, poverty, poor education, provision of health services and sewerage systems. If they get employment, the migrants usually work in the informal sector because of their lack of skills and education and are stuck with the 'dirty' jobs. Family relationships are under threat because of long-term separations for work, or overcrowding and poverty. Drugs, gangs and crime also flourish in the informal economy that survives with corruption at many levels.

In developing countries employment conditions in informal employment and informal jobs, child labour, and slavery/bonded labour are of major importance. Within informal employment there are few protections for workers such as regulations about minimal wages, hours of work, conditions of employment and occupational health and safety. Those who are least able to resist, children and women are heavily represented in those who are involved in forced labour. Throughout the world 317 million children aged between 5-17 years work and 218 are child labourers, and many, 126 million, are involved in hazardous work. The current estimate is that there are about 28 million salves and 5.7 million children in forced or bonded labour in the world (EMCONET 2007, 16). The children in forced labour suffer from the effects of the work environment, for example, cramped conditions, poor lighting, heavy lifting etc and also suffer from the lack of normal development process of childhood for example, family support, education, shelter and peer childhood relationships.

6. Recent research

6.1 Developing countries employment and health

There are two pieces of research that I have conducted recently that relate to the employment and health. The first was conducted with my colleague Dr Leigh Lehane in 2006. It was a small study in primary health care in rural Thailand: *Towards realising primary health care for the rural poor in Thailand: health policy in action,* and demonstrates the nature of health issues generally for the rural population but in particular it demonstrates the problems of employee health and the lack of awareness of the toxicity of pesticides in developing countries. Because of the small scale of this study the results can only be taken as indicative. This work was accepted for publication after having been peer reviewed but was withdrawn from publication by the editor because of its political nature.

(We acknowledge Thai workers and colleagues for their help, kindness and generosity; the University of New England, for a University Research Grant; and Nakhon Ratchasima Provincial Health Office for accommodation and transport.)

Introduction

In 2001 Thailand established Universal Health Coverage (UHC) to provide primary health care (PHC) through its network of 9,738 primary care units (PCUs) (sometimes also called health centres) to make health care accessible for uninsured Thais (including about 40 million rural people). UHC (known as the '30 Baht Scheme') meant that, for patients, the cost of medical and hospital treatment was 30 baht per episode of care (Wibulpolprasert 2002). In October 2006, General Surayud Chulanont, the current Prime Minister of Thailand and Head of the Interim Government, abolished the 30 baht fee and made the health care program free (The Nation, 2006).

PHC services in Thailand provide treatment for common illnesses and injuries, health promotion, disease prevention and control and rehabilitation. PHC refers to first contact, continuous, comprehensive and coordinated care (Ministry of Public Health, 2001) (Starfield 1994).

PHC for Thailand's rural poor has been problematic because of a shortage of rural medical practitioners (Wibulpolprasert and Pengpaibon 2003) and challenges raised by recent epidemics, such as avian influenza, SARS and HIV/AIDS(Beaglehold 2004, World Health Organisation 2003).

The authors, comprising the research team, looked at what PHC was being done, and how well it was being done, by one rural PCU. The aim was to provide Thai stakeholders, among whom were executives, senior provincial health officers and academics, with a report that would help them implement strategies to improve PHC throughout rural Thailand.

Methods

The authors evaluated the delivery of PHC at one PCU in Nakhon Ratchasima ('Khorat') Province, Thailand. The research design is best described as a case study. During the course of the study we were immersed in the life of the PCU for one month and lived in Provincial Health Services accommodation for that period.

The case study PCU was located about 250 km north-east of Bangkok and was chosen by the Thai stakeholders in collaboration with the researchers because it was considered to be representative of most PCUs throughout rural Thailand. Thai stakeholders included the Provincial Chief Medical Officer; Dean of Public Health from a rural university in another province; Community Hospital Director of the District Hospital; other provincial health officers, including the Provincial Chief Development Officer in charge of Training and Research; and staff of the selected PCU and a Thai health professional/interpreter.

The population served by the case study PCU was comprised of 2800 villagers, most of whom were poor (Jitsanguan, 2001) earning a seasonal income of about 3000 baht (around A$100) a month as labourers and small-scale farmers (National Economic and Social Development Board 2004). The nearest private doctor's clinic was 14 km from the PCU, but it was economically beyond the reach of most villagers. PCUs throughout the district were supported by a 30-bed referral hospital which served a total population of 27,616 people from 46 villages. Selected characteristics of the case study PCU and the district hospital are shown in Table 3.

According to the Community Hospital Director of the District Hospital in which the research was conducted, the main causes of death for the population served by the case study PCU were:

• Heart/circulatory disease (151.96/100,000 persons)
• HIV/AIDS and other infections (81.3/100,000 persons)
• Cancer (63.6/100,000 persons)
• Accidents (42.4/100,000 persons).

The leading causes of morbidity were respiratory disease, digestive problems, musculo-skeletal problems, infections and circulatory diseases.

The questions used to guide the evaluation were:

• What PHC is provided by the PCU?
• How well is PHC delivered by the PCU?

During the process of data collection, we sought to elicit whether the care provided by the PCU was relevant and appropriate for the patient; done well; made available in a timely manner to patients who needed it; continuous with other care and care providers; performed in a safe, efficient caring manner; and respectful of the patient (Gilpatrick 1999).

	PCU	District Hospital
Nurses	3 nurses: 1 nurse manager 1 general nurse (4 years training) 1 public health nurse (2 years training)	23 nurses (training details not available)
Doctors	1 doctor, 5 hours a month	4 full-time doctors
Dentists	1 dental assistant, 3 hours a month	2 full-time dentists
Pharmacists	1 pharmacist, 3 hours a month	3 full-time pharmacists
Additional experts	None	15 (e.g., health promotion officer, radiologist)
Population served	2,800 people from5 villages rural poor small scale farmers serving geographical area of 30km2	27,616 people from 46 villages rural poor small scale farmers serving geographical area of 200km2
Capacity	No inpatients beds 6,000 outpatients consultation per year	30 inpatient beds 38,000 outpatients consultations per year
Facilities	Two story concrete building Motor cycle for nurses providing community work	Single –level building with dormitory for inpatient accommodation; outpatients; radiology; laboratory; administrative areas; conference facilities; cars and ambulances.

Table 3. Selected characteristics of the case study Primary Care Unit and the associated District Hospital

Starfield's approach to evaluating the quality of primary health care (Starfield 1998) informed the study variables and methods of data-gathering (Table 2). The latter were primarily qualitative, and included interviewing, focus groups, observations, and documentary and photographic analysis. Data were collected in field notes, and when focus groups and interviews were conducted they were then translated into English.

By accompanying the PCU staff on all their duties and using Kemmis and McTaggart's 'spiral of self-reflective cycles', (2000) we reflected daily with the PCU staff on the data gathered. Each afternoon the researchers (with their field notes) and the PCU staff would discuss the patients seen in the clinic that day. These discussions involved examination of patient records in family folders. The family folder is the primary health record file in the PCU and it contains brief health information of all family members, a genogram, family members' general characteristics, major health problems of each, and progress notes on treatment (Sennun, Suwannapong, Howteerakul, and Pacheun 2006). Questions arising from these discussions provoked subsequent investigations. Every evening the researchers reflected on the data gathered and prepared questions to be answered the following day with the help of the PCU staff.

Thai stakeholders participated in two reflective focus groups (Table 3), each of about three hours duration; one in the first week of the research and a second at the end, when an interim report was presented and discussed. Both focus groups were facilitated by the principal researcher, and a Thai interpreter, who was also a health professional, was used throughout the project.

Starfield's unique attributes and appropriate sources of evidence[1]		Application to this study
Unique attributes of PHC* and process elements/study variables***	Sources of evidence**	Methods used in this study
First contact care: Accessibility of the service and the extent of actual use of the service Process element of performance in regard to first contact care: utilisation.	Program design: hours of availability; accessibility to public transport; provision of care without requirements for payment in advance; facilities for handicapped; after-hours arrangements; ease of making appointments; and absence of language and other cultural barriers.	Program design was accessed by: interviews with staff and local health officials; taped focus groups with stakeholders; observations of daily activities of PCU over one month; observations of patient care; interviews with patients and villagers; review of charts of patients seen each day; home visits; attendance at governance meetings.
Longitudinality: Person focused contact over time (involves the extent of provider-consumer contact for all but referred care) Process elements of performance in regard to longitudinality: population eligibility; patient identification with a particular provider.	Review of patient lists and interviews with patients about the regularity of their contact for disease management; management of signs and symptoms; administration(need for certification of illness and health) test results; need for and return from consultation for secondary level care; and prescription of drugs and other therapies.	Reviews of patients claims/costs under Universal Health Coverage (UHC); receipts; records (family folders); clinical and management documents of PCU. Attendance at presentations of 1) structure of health services in the District; and 2) Structure of health services at PCU.
Comprehensiveness: Primary health care services to meet the common needs of the consumer over time. Process elements of performance in regard to comprehensiveness: problem recognition; diagnosis; management and assessment; knowledge of patient's social profile; recognition of psychological problems; attitude towards and knowledge of preventive and psychological needs.	Recognition of the range of activities the system is designed to handle.	Documents reviewed: agenda of April meeting of the Contracting unit of the PHC Board; avian influenza simulation rapid response team exercise; after action review of above; checklist of yearly review of PCU activities; health education review document, which every household had to complete; health survey for diabetes and hypertension;

Coordination: Health –related services and information brought to bear on patient care. Process elements of performance in regard to coordination; recognition of information from visits elsewhere; documentation of medication and compliance; problem lists/problem-orientated medical records; preventive care.	Patient records and interviews; seeking information about prior visits; the organized system of referral and retrieval of information about the results of referral	list of disabled people; antenatal record book; personal health record book. Review of clinical information system: methods, nature of, frequency of, and type of communication.

1. Starfield B. Primary care: balancing health needs, services and technology. New York: Oxford University Press; 1998 (*p. 29-30; **p. 282; ***p. 255-261)

Table 4. Conceptual framework used to guide study variables and data collection methods

The standards and protocols against which the process elements were evaluated were those of the Australian College of Rural and Remote Medicine (1997) and the Royal Australian College of General Practitioners, which were familiar to the Thai stakeholders and the researchers. The principal researcher was familiar with agricultural chemical management strategies as a member of the Safety Institute of Australia (SIA) and the Global Occupational Health Network (GOHNET).

The research proposal was approved by the Human Research Ethics Committee of the University of New England, Armidale, Australia. Nakhon Ratchasima Province Health Services accepted the Australian Ethics Committee approval to proceed. Information sheets for participants and consent forms were translated into Thai and the Thai interpreter ensured that the informants understood their part in the research process.

Results

First contact care

Accessibility and utilisation of the services provided by the PCU were influenced by the lack of public transport. Most patients walked to the clinic, others came on the back of trucks, or on motorcycles carrying up to four people (including children). Handicapped or elderly patients were sometimes wheeled along the side of the road in barrows. The District Hospital reimbursed a local villager for the use of his truck in emergencies, when it was used as an ambulance.

Thais are registered at the PCU nearest where they live for purposes of UHC, but people sometimes sought care elsewhere. This occurred for reasons of privacy (e.g. women seeking abortions), convenience (e.g. seasonal workers who became injured in the district), or lack of confidence in the staff of the PCU at which they were registered. Clinical reports were not sent back to the home PCUs of such patients.

When a person was referred to a hospital, or for specialist services in Bangkok, the contact between the patient and staff at the PCU was disrupted. This was because the PCU staff did not receive timely advice on the diagnosis, treatment or prognosis that was made elsewhere, nor were they consulted on what part they could take in the patient's treatment or rehabilitation.

FOCUS GROUP 1		FOCUS GROUP 2	
Participants	Procedures	Participants	Procedures
• PCU staff: nurse manager, general trained nurse, public health trained nurse • Provincial Chief Medical Officer • Community Hospital Director of District Hospital • Nurse Manager of PCU at District Hospital • District Chief Health Officer (Public Health) ☐ Health professional/interpreter	Topics discussed: • The nature of the research project, and what was required of the participants. All questions were answered and suggestions from participants recorded.	• PCU staff: nurse manager, general trained nurse, public health trained nurse • Provincial Chief Medical Officer • Dean of Public Health* • Community Hospital Director • Nurse Manager of PCU at District Hospital • District Chief Health Officer • Chief of Local Government • Head of Administration in Local Government • Assistant Provincial Chief Medical Officer • Provincial Chief Development Officer in charge of training and research and • Deputy Provincial Chief Development Officer (training and research) ☐ Health professional/interpreter	Topics discussed: • The research process • The research findings, conclusions and recommendations. Stakeholders' opinions and discussion points, including possible means of implementation of recommendations, were recorded.

*At the time of the focus group 2 this informant had resigned from this position temporarily and was elected Senator of the Thai legislature. After the coup of 2006, he returned to the position of Dean of Public Health.

Table 5. Focus group participants and procedures

Thais registered at other PCUs were welcomed at the PCU if they chose to come there. Elderly people attended for repeat prescriptions and minor illnesses. Patients with minor injuries came for dressings, because some of them could not afford to buy bandages or antiseptic.

The usual number of patients per day was between 10 and 20. On antenatal days, the PCU staff attended to between 20 and 30 women. When the doctor, pharmacist and dental assistant visited the unit, the number of patients swelled to between 60 and 80. Whereas the nurses sometimes spent up to an hour on a consultation, the doctor spent about five minutes with each person. The dental assistant bought a mobile dental chair to the PCU and treated about 15 people during each three hour session; extracting teeth and prescribing antibiotics for abscesses. The dentist at the District Hospital performed more difficult procedures (e.g., fillings).

Longitudinality

Measurement of 'longitudinality' relates to who in the population is eligible to receive PHC from this PCU, and how exclusive that eligibility is. This is linked to the concept of identification of the patient with the provider over time.

Thais are registered at the PCU nearest where they live for purposes of UHC, but people sometimes sought care elsewhere. This occurred for reasons of privacy (e.g. women seeking abortions), convenience (e.g. seasonal workers who became injured in the district), or lack of confidence in the staff of the PCU at which they were registered. Clinical reports were not sent back to the home PCUs of such patients.

When a person was referred to a hospital, or for specialist services in Bangkok, the contact between the patient and staff at the PCU was disrupted. This was because the PCU staff did not receive timely advice on the diagnosis, treatment or prognosis that was made elsewhere, nor were they consulted on what part they could take in the patient's treatment or rehabilitation.

Comprehensiveness

As indicated in Table 2, measures of the comprehensiveness of PHC services deal with: problem recognition; diagnosis, management and reassessment; knowledge of patients' social profile; recognition of psychological problems; and attitudes towards and knowledge of preventive and psychological needs. The following examples demonstrate the complex nature of the problems presenting to the PCU and the inadequacy of some diagnoses by PCU staff:

1. While waiting to see the doctor on his monthly visit to the PCU, middle-aged women chewed betel nuts as they talked together. When these women went to the dentist for extraction the first author noted what appeared to be palatal leucoplakia (precancerous slowly developing change in the mucous membrane) and gum disease. The same women complained to the doctor of longstanding insomnia and abdominal pain. They were diagnosed with 'insomnia' and 'dyspepsia', and given sedatives and antacids. It was neither considered nor recorded that the women were betel-nut chewers, although they openly enjoyed the habit as they waited to be seen.

2. A cluster of four people, one man and three women, presented over a period of 18 hours with fatigue, headaches, dizziness, itchy skin, blurred vision and sore eyes. On examination they all exhibited very low blood pressure. The diagnosis was 'weakness', and they were treated with vitamin B complex and analgesics without advice on the possible cause of the condition or means of preventing its recurrence. We found that these patients were all agricultural workers who did not use personal protective equipment when spraying chemicals in the hours before presentation at the PCU. The most severely affected woman had a blood pressure of 90/60. The researchers and PCU staff followed up this woman the next day at her second worksite and found that her blood pressure had returned to normal.

3. Six people, four men and two children, presented with cuts and deep lacerations to the feet and lower legs. These injuries, including those of the children, occurred at work, and were caused by knives, machinery or broken glass. The villagers either went without shoes entirely or wore rubber 'thongs' or 'flip-flops'. Although antibiotics were used, healing was delayed because the staff were not permitted to take swabs for microbiological diagnosis and sensitivity testing; dressings were cheap and not water-

proof; and the local water was not clean. Preventive strategies (e.g. encouragement to wear shoes) were not considered. Two of the men smelt of alcohol and their regular and excessive alcohol intake was known to the PCU staff. The latter did not comment or try to intervene about the alcohol abuse, explaining to us that it was a private matter for the patient.

We observed that many older patients presented regularly with the same complaints, and received the same combination of medications, without their clinical data being reviewed periodically for reassessment. One woman with diabetes, who had multiple PCU service contacts, several inpatient stays in the District Hospital and ten doctor consultations, had no reassessment or enquiry about her lack of compliance with control of blood sugar.

Coordination

Measures of coordination included: retrieval of health information about consultations conducted elsewhere; documentation of medication and compliance; problem lists/ problem-orientated medical records; and population and individual preventive care. Coordination was problematic at the PCU in many ways.

There were instances of children with congenital disorders and blindness who had been referred to specialists, but no information accompanied the family on return, or was sent back to the PCU. The PCU did not have a landline telephone. The staff relied for communication on mobile technology, erratic internet connections, and personal travel (mainly by motorcycle). They did not have ready access to supervision about problem cases.

There were several tools used in the PCU for documentation of patients' records: the family folder; a personal records book; and an antenatal care records book. Information on the social, occupational and economic history of the patient, together with the history of clinical or surgical contact, was not gathered together in one file. Primary data such as those contained in laboratory reports were transcribed by hand, with the possibility of introducing errors. The personal records book and the antenatal care records book were used to a variable extent by the community.

The PCU staff showed some natural reserve in talking of 'moral' or 'private' matters (e.g. alcoholism, drug addiction and HIV/AIDS) although, on enquiry from us, they were generally well aware of patients' problems. This was not just discretion in front of the researchers: such issues tended to be ignored, not being discussed in interviews with patients or recorded in family folders. The Thai interpreter would return at a later stage by himself without the 'farangs' (Thai word meaning foreigners) and discuss some of these culturally sensitive issues fully with the staff to gain a better understanding of their approach in these matters.

Statistics on HIV/AIDS were collated by local government officials. Testing was done confidentially at the District Hospital and provision for income support was available through local government. However, information that existed on the incidence of HIV/AIDS and its prevention was not freely disseminated. Condoms were available on request as part of the HIV/AIDS program of the Ministry of Public Health and we were told PCU staff advertised this in villages. However, although AIDS was the fifth most common cause of death in the district, only one man asked for condoms during the period of our research. In antenatal care, women were given the choice of an HIV test, but, as they had to pay themselves, only about half took up the offer.

Medicines were handed out liberally after each consultation. These included antibiotics, anti-inflammatories, antifungals, antihistamines, analgesics, antacids and sedatives. No record of the medications received by the family was included in their folder. Some medications (e.g. digitalis) could not be dispensed by the nurses, even for repeat prescriptions, and writing out repeat prescriptions took up a large part of the time of the doctor's monthly visit to the PCU.

Discussion

Principal findings

The PCU can act as a 'gatekeeper' to specialist health services in the District Hospital, protecting the patient from unnecessary medical treatment and limiting access to high-cost medical services (Franks, Clancy, Nutting 1992) There is a trade-off between freedom of the patient to choose and operational efficiency of health services management. Both the transport arrangements and the lack of advanced-level medical functions (e.g. reassessments, clarifying differential diagnoses, supervision and training, and complex case management) at the PCU did not allow it to act in a gatekeeper role. The PCU could not provide comprehensive care for the patients over time because of a lack of diagnostic skills of the PCU staff; and lack of access to direct supervision by the PCU staff.

PHC differs from secondary and tertiary care because of the lack of differentiation of the problems that present in the primary care setting (Starfield 1998). The women with insomnia, decayed teeth and dyspepsia are examples of poor problem recognition and staff-selective attitudes towards preventive health because betel nut is the most widely used stimulant in the developing world and is associated commonly with dental decay, oral cancers, insomnia, stomach discomfort and intestinal cancers (International Agency for Research on Cancer Monographs 2004). Betel-nut chewing was considered by the PCU staff to be the private business of the patients and not part of their responsibility as health professionals. Similarly the presenting symptoms of the agricultural workers were not considered work-related. However, such symptoms are commonly attributed to agricultural chemical toxicity. Acute chemical toxicity is the major problem arising from the use of pesticides in the developing world (Jeyaratnam 1999). Community preventive strategies were not developed from an awareness of local need because preventive health programs were decided nationally. Despite the weakness of problem definition, the health data from the PCU went on to become statistics in district, provincial and national health databases.

PCU staff were not included in ongoing health interventions initiated by other services, with the result that patients could not go to the PCU for informed follow-up care. Because these patients were poor and not medically literate, this was a deficiency in the quality of health services available to them. While the family folder is important institutionally and traditionally because it conveys a family focus, it had shortcomings as a medical record as it was not adapted to the mobility and privacy of the rural people.

Strengths and weaknesses of the study

The strengths and weaknesses of this study are those associated with the case study design. A strength of the design is the intense focus on a single case (here it was the rural PCU). Such an approach has the potential to provide new insights into complex organisational issues that may be used to build theory (Bryman 2004). This research was further strengthened by the use of Starfield's conceptual framework (1998) and the involvement of PCU staff and Thai stakeholders in the final stages of data analysis and interpretation. The main weakness of the design is that the results are not able to be generalised to the relevant population; a problem of external validity. Despite these known limitations, Thai stakeholders accepted the findings presented in an interim report as a true account of PHC at that case study PCU, and considered them to be applicable to other rural PHC settings in Thailand.

Policy and practice implications

As a result of our study, it was recommended that health professionals in rural PCUs in Thailand would benefit from:

- clinical supervision with specific, regular and close attention from experts;
- provision of timely/appropriate/accurate information to use for patient care;
- training programs for clinical, community, occupational and management skills-development at the PHC level; and
- authority to prioritise services for the disabled and aged through the development of a health advocacy role for the PCU Manager.

With a community approach in PHC as recommended by the World Health Organization (WHO) in 2003, PCU staff should be trained to recognise and institute control measures for occupational illnesses; conduct assessments of mental status, and provide supportive counselling for alcohol and drug abuse; teach children to floss and brush teeth regularly; and provide education on HIV/AIDS prevention. Thailand has one of the highest pharmaceutical drug consumption rates per capita in the world, (Cohen 1989, Filmer, Hammer, and Pritchett, 1997) a fact that indicates a strongly embedded bias towards curative rather than preventive medicine. Improving the efficiency of the supply and use of drugs is one management system change that would reduce costs substantially. Health initiatives to provide trained health professionals are needed where public health infrastructure and occupational and environmental health are poorly developed and the community lives in or near poverty. Research into methods and processes of collaboration and communication between primary and secondary care needs to be carried out in order to integrate community, PCU and hospital services.

Conclusion

This process evaluation of one PCU in rural Thailand five years after UHC was introduced in 2001 was undertaken to provide Thai stakeholders with recommendations to improve the quality of PHC within current resource constraints. The evaluation concluded that improvements in the performance of PHC in rural Thailand could be made so that resource use could be maximised.

Thai stakeholders contributed to the evaluation and accepted the interim report as a true account of PHC at the case study PCU. They considered the recommendations appropriate for application in this setting and possibly other rural PHC settings in Thailand and indicated that they intended to implement the recommendations in the study province

6.2 Developed countries, employment and mental illness

The second piece of research that I conducted has been published in the journal, Higher Education Research and Development, and is titled: *How social relationships influence academic health in the 'enterprise university': an insight into productivity of knowledge workers*. This is an important article from my thesis research that is available in a book: *The health that workers want*.

This research highlights some important aspects of contemporary employment. The employment relations, employment conditions and working conditions in developed countries impact on employees' mental health because of the social relationships in the work environment. When employees feel the psychological contract is not balanced they respond by withdrawing their efforts.

Social relations in the work place

Downsizing is the most common form of rationalising business operations by reducing salaries and expenses. Leigh and Mayhew (2002:344) report that 10% of workers suffer a stress-related or depressive illness each year and there are increased proportions of stressed workers in organisations undergoing large-scale restructuring, and that stress contributes to 30% of all work-related illnesses. Downsizing produces two types of problem that influence health according to the Demand–Control–Support theory. First, there is increased workload because of reduced staff and second, there is loss of support as staff networks are disrupted by redundancies or redeployment of staff. The combination of high expectations and low support is frequently associated with dissatisfaction and ill health according to Karasek's (1979) Demand–Control–Support theory. Employees are affected by the way work is constituted, constructed and managed, and in service industries, work is a socially determined activity and the social nature of work has positive and negative benefits for health and productivity. Putnam's 'social capital' (2000:326) is a group level construct and refers to social connectedness through these social relationships, and according to Putnam, is one of the most powerful determinants of well being. Social capital is a metaphor for performance advantage obtained by social network development as a function of social structure (Burt 2000:346).

The employee–employer relationship has been conceptualised in the psychological contract since Barnard in 1938 and refers to the exchange of implicit and explicit factors that bind the parties in the relationship. Rousseau (1995:7) comments on the difficulty of reestablishing balances between the contributions that employees make and the inducements that organisations offer to employees when those balances are disturbed. Employees actively change what they offer to the organisation if they perceive that the inducements (i.e. material and social rewards) are not appropriate, particularly in relation to their health and wellbeing. The nature of the employer–employee relationship is important in shaping the work culture and the dynamism of this relationship is demonstrated in relation to critical health events when employees change their behaviour.

Employee behavioural responses, particularly to restructuring in organisational and industrial changes show two main forms. Individualistic employees try to cope by detaching intellectually and/or physically from the organisation and 'working to rule', while in the other response employees try to change the workplace from within. This detachment from the organisation is also a detachment from social networks at work. In its extreme form this detachment is called 'presenteeism' which means that the employees comes to work but actually does not contribute much to productivity. Not only does each response require a personal struggle on the part of the followers, the existence of the two responses in the one workplace creates division among the employees and there is a risk of disunity, dissent and multiple purposes within the work culture.

The rationale of employers supporting restructures and their proposed view of its implementation are not consistent with the reality that unfolds for employees. The rhetoric of employers is that employees will be listened to, workload will not change, and it will all be for the best, but in fact, employees find that their comments are ignored, or worse, regarded as divisive, and the workload increases.

The four issues that define and differentiate types of stress are: the sense of control the employee have over the work situation; the balance that exists between the work and home domains in the employees life; the perception of the effort put into work and the rewards received for that effort; and finally the relationships at work with fellow workers, supervisors and managers. The first three issues are more important to differentiate workplace stress as productive or counterproductive. Whereas the last issue, that is, relationships at work, is more significant for the pervasive and formless systemic stress that is felt at the level of the workgroup.

Productive workplace stress is associated with intellectual stimulation and accomplishment, and counterproductive workplace stress is associated with negative states such as limitation and burden. These individual perspectives of workplace stress are positivist representations of the 'reality' of the employer–employee relationship at work. Ways of thinking about workplace stress are culture bound in this relationship. However, recognising systemic stress challenges the limitations of this epistemiology and ontology. The third type of workplace stress is more diffuse and is associated with lower levels of trust in the organisation and is a social reality rather than and individual reality. With social or post-modern relativism this additional and systemic stress is cultural bound, socially conditioned, historically relative and contextual; it is as Scheurich's (1997: 34) states 'a political struggle'. The broad issues involved in coping with workplace stress relate to the active response of employees to workplace stress, the different categories of staff affected and their evolving experience of the workplace operated at the level of the individual, workgroup and the organisation. The health effects of workplace stress are described as minor and major physical and mental illnesses affecting the individual and a more generalised reduction in the quality of employees' lives. Stress in the workplace is summarised in below.

- Productive stress
  - stress is productive when there is the successful application of the individual employees abilities
  - work tasks are associated with intellectual stimulation and work is a challenge that is achievable
  - central issues for the individual are: a sense of control about how and when to do work; rewards are appropriate to efforts extended; the employee's skills are fit for the work duties
  - employment contract is mutually rewarding, characterised by trust
- Counterproductive stress
  - stress is counterproductive when work is a burden to endure because tasks constrain the employee and limit the sense of achievement
  - origin of counterproductive stress is quantitative and qualitative work overload
  - central issues for the individual are: decreased control and imbalance between effort extended and reward received
  - employment contract is not satisfactory to employees and they feel exploited
- Systemic stress
  - stress is systemic because it operates at the level of the workgroup and is associated with negativity in the social processes of the work environment
  - origins of systemic stress are competitive adjustments of organisations in market economies

- employer–employee master narrative is positivist and acknowledges competition but does not acknowledge the impact of competition on social processes at work
- work activities are made harder
- central issues for the workgroup and organisation are the development of individualism and the fragmentation of social relationships
- employment contract is strategically managed by both employers who want knowledge workers with flexibility, and employees who want continuous financial security though employment with one or a series of employers
- Broad issues in coping
  - employees are active in coping with workplace stress
  - different categories of staff react differently to stress
  - responses to workplace stress at different levels, that is, individuals, workgroups and organisations to workplace stress are dynamic, changing over time.
- Health effects
  - employees suffer minor and major physical and mental illness
  - reduced quality of life can occur

Bullying in the workplace is the failure management to shape workplace relationships in a constructive manner. The phenomena of bullying, in its obvious form is associated with persistent insults, offensive remarks, persistent criticism, personal and even physical abuse. In its subtle form bully consists of excluding or isolating the victim from his/her peer group or excluding them from information and/or appropriate interactions and opportunities in the workplace. The exact frequency of bullying is hard to determine but it is generally more common that employers like to state Einarsen et al (2003). In Australia the federal health and Safety regulator Comcare said that workplace bullying is on par with workplace stress as the main causes of serious mental stress claims (Griffiths, 2011).

Employees who suffer mental illness are disadvantaged compared to employees with physical illnesses for two reasons. Firstly the nature of mental illness is such that it rarely starts suddenly. There is a gradual deterioration in wellbeing particularly with depression, and with treatment there is a gradual recovery. The gradual nature of the onset and recovery means that the employee is likely to be at work and not performing at his/her best. This is usually hidden, and fellow workmates cover and do what is necessary to protect their colleague, or if it is obvious the lower performance is viewed critically. The burden of hiding the depression-illness is an additional problem for the employee as workplaces generally are not sympathetic or knowledge about the true nature of the cycle of depression and its impact on the persons' performance.

7. Future research

Employment and mental illness is an important area for future research. These include:
1. What are the optimal social networks and social supports for employees and employee groups in different situations and how are these matched?
   There is not a universal social network or support that is beneficial to all employees in every circumstance. For example, employees living alone and near retirement have different social needs from the workplace than young employees with children who are just entering the workplace. Tailoring support to the particular mix of employees would ensure the most beneficial effect for their health in the most efficient manner.

2. What are the mechanisms of action of social relationships on health?
    Rutter (1985:316) suggests that the protective processes of social relationships may act
    in several ways: (1) by reducing exposure to risk by groups being more cohesive; (2) by
    reducing negative consequences of exposure to risk; (3) by developing employees'
    resilience through increased self-esteem and self-worth; and (4) by developing
    enhanced adaptive behaviour through the opportunities for better outcomes at critical
    turning points in employees' lives. The mechanism of action of social relationships on
    health may also be determined by the nature of the risk that the individual within the
    group is exposed to. Greater knowledge of the buffering and transmitting effects of
    social relationships would increase our understanding of disease patterns.

3. How can the concept of stress be clarified to incorporate the reality of compounding
    factors, variable timeframes, vulnerability and resilience and assessment of outcomes?
    Research in the empirical world of work needs to consider compounding factors,
    variable timeframes and lengths of exposure and latency periods for illness onset. These
    issues represent the reality of risks at work in contrast to the injury model with its
    isolated exposure to a noxious environment causing an immediate illness. The injury
    model is applied inappropriately to illness and disease at work.

4. What are constructive human resource interventions with organisational change?
    With organisational change being common, human resource management needs to
    follow the process through so that employees who are retained in employment are
    better able to manage. Human resource interventions would be constructive if they
    prevented harm to employees and sustained productivity after the restructure.

5. What are the short-term and long-term influences of electronic communication systems
    and new technology on the socialisation process?
    Electronic communication and new technology are pervasive in everyday life and at
    work in particular. The speed of information transfer is obvious but the effect on
    accepted behavioural patterns and activities of employees is less obvious.

6. What are the effects of telework on employee health and organisational productivity?
    The various forms of telework are increasingly used by organisations to attract staff that
    they would otherwise not be able to employ. Telework also removes the need to
    provide office space and other facilities for staff. There is increased need however for
    communication and monitoring systems to ensure that outcomes are achieved.
    Additionally, for complex deliverables the coordination functions of a project manager
    are needed to bring together the outputs of employees with disparate skills connected
    by communication systems. With extensive use of telework as an organisational
    strategy for competitive advantage, the skills of the management and the well being of
    the employees need to be reviewed because telework is a significant departure from the
    familiar workplace where employers and employees are housed together.

7. What are the health effects of mobility and short-term contracts on executives, and what
    are their mechanisms of action?
    Nowadays the vulnerability of lower paid workers to changes in employment contracts
    is seen in the increasing use of part time staff, short-term contracts and other strategies
    to allow the organisation flexibility to hire staff with the skills that are needed at the
    time, and terminate those employees when they are not needed.
    At the other end of the spectrum, executives too are accepting short-term contracts.
    However, compensation would be made in the contract for the executive for the risk of
    unemployment between contracts. Nevertheless, the health effects of mobility and

short-term contracts are important considerations for this group of executive employees.

8.   What are the health effects of quality employment on women? In dealing with workplace stress, how do women's coping styles differ from those of men, particularly when they are in the same industry?

It is important to specify as carefully as possible what factors influence health. The notion of quality employment has merit because it implies some freedom over the work situation that is not there with low quality employment. When summarising the literature in the area of workplace stress, Langan-Fox (1998:273) recognised coping styles being influenced by gender. In the qualitative data this research shows some differences between married women and men in their adjustment to work, but that adjustment is hinged around the needs of children. Women without children and women who are single parents are not identified in the qualitative data. Further clarification of the issues that are involved here, (that is, responsibility for children, financial resources in the home and living as a single parent) would be helpful to identify the impact of gender on employee health.

9.   What is the optimal mix of values for employee health and organisational outcomes and how can that mix be achieved?

The values of the stakeholders embedded in the employer–employee relationships are vary. Some values, such as competitiveness, support profit over health, whereas other values, for example, sustainability, indicate a long-term view with profit being reconciled with social justice. The present employer–employee relationship is dominated by profit generating values and policies and practices that flow from these values are utilitarian and individualistic in nature. Being aware of this starting point and trying to change these values is more useful than trying to negotiate within the present employer–employee relationship. The optimum mix of the various stakeholders' values would ensure both organisational profit and employee health are achieved. This mix would produce greater flexibility with the utilitarian and ontological variation in individualism–collectivism dimension in the employer–employee relationship.

8. Conclusions

In this chapter employment and its link to the burden of mental illness, has been traced in its theoretical and practical aspects. Employment is a major factor in the genesis of ill health. In developing countries employment is on the whole agricultural and the major hazards are chemical poisoning and physical injury. Recent research in rural Thailand is presented to highlight these factors.

In developed countries where service industries are predominant the main health problems are those related to stress and bullying with the erosion of employment conditions. Recent research highlights the complex nature of stress at work and its impact on employees. The employer-employee master narrative dominates work and is responsible for social relationships at work that bear heavily on stress situations and create the environment for bullying.

Employment and mental illness is a rich area for future research and many factors that bear on employment conditions and work conditions need to be researched to find ways to improve work for the heath and well being of employees. The employer-employee master narrative will be influenced by increasing awareness of the impact on productivity of many of the poor work arrangements that harm employee's mental health.

9. References

Aarts, L. J. M. & De Jong, P. R. 1992, Economic Aspects of Disability Behaviour, Elsevier Science Publishers, Amsterdam.

Acheson Report, 1998, Independent Inquiry into Inequalities in Health, The Stationery Office, London.

Allvin, M. & Aronsson, G. 2003, 'The Future of Work Environment Reforms: Does the Concept of Work Environment apply within the New Economy?' International Journal of Health Services, vol. 33, no. 1, pp. 99–111.

American Network of Health Promoting Universities 2002, [Online], Available: http://www. ahcnet.org/programs/leadership/anhpu.php, [Accessed 19 June 2004].

Anderson, D. R., Serxner, S. A. & Gold, D.B. 2001, 'Conceptual Framework, Critical Questions, and Practical Challenges in conducting Research on the Financial Impact of Worksite Health Promotion', American Journal of Health Promotion, vol. 15 no. 5, pp. 281–295.

Anthony, P. 1994, Managing Culture, Open University Press, Buckingham.

Armour, R. A. 1987, 'Academic Burnout: Faculty responsibility and institutional climate', New Directions for Teaching and Learning vol. 29, pp. 3–11.

Aronsson, G., Gustafsson, K. & Dallner, M. 2000, 'Sick but yet at work. An empirical study of sickness presenteeism', J Epidemiology and Community Health, vol. 54, pp. 502–509.

Australian Bureau of Statistics, 2000, Labour Mobility, Australia, Catalogue No. 6209.0, AGPS,

Australian Bureau of Statistics, 2000, Working Arrangements, Australia, AGPS, Canberra.

Australian Bureau of Statistics, 2003, Australian Demographic Statistics, Catalogue No. 3101.0, AGPS, Canberra.

Australian Bureau of Statistics, 2003, Australian Social Trends: Health, Risk Factors, Health Risk Factors among Adults, AGPS, Canberra.

Australian College of Rural and Remote Medicine. 1997, Primary curriculum for rural and remote medicine. 2nd ed. Brisbane: Australian College of Rural and Remote Medicine; Available from: http://www.acrrm.org.au (Accessed 15/1/07.)

Australian Institute of Health and Welfare 2000, Australia's Health in 2000: The Seventh Biennial Report of the Australian Institute of Health and Welfare. AGPS, Canberra.

Australian Institute of Health and Welfare 2001, National Drug Strategy Household Survey, AGPS, Canberra.

Australian Research Council 2003, Description of Designated National Research Priorities and Associated Priority Goals, AGPS, Canberra.

Australian Research Council, 2004, RFCD, SEO and ANZSIC Codes 2003. AGPS, Canberra.

Avison, W. R. & Gotlib, I. H. 1994, 'Future Prospects for Stress Research', in Stress and Mental Health: Contemporary issues and prospects for the future, eds W.R. Avison & I.H. Gotlib, Plenum Press, New York, pp. 317–332.

Barnard, C. I. 1938, The Functions of the Executive, Harvard University Press, Cambridge.

Bates, E. & Linder-Pelz, S. 1987, Health Care Issues, Allen & Unwin, Sydney.

Baum, F. 1999, 'Social capital: Is it good for your health? Issues for a public health agenda', J Epidemiology and Community Health, vol. 53, pp. 195–196.

Bauman, L. J., Stein, R. E. K & Ireys, H.T. 1991, 'Reinventing fidelity: The transfer of social technology amongst settings', American Journal of Community Psychology, vol. 19, pp. 619–639.

Bayer, R. 1986, 'Notifying Workers at Risk: Politics of the Right-to-Know', American Journal of Public Health, vol. 76 no. 11, pp. 1352–1356.

Beaglehole R. 2004, Global public health: a new era. Oxford: Oxford University Press.

Beck, U. 1992, Risk Society: Towards a New Modernity, Sage Publications, London.

Berger, Y. 1999, 'Why hasn't it changed on the Shopfloor?' in Occupational Health and Safety in Australia: Industry, Public Sector, and Small Business, eds C. Mayhew & C. Peterson, Allen & Unwin, Sydney, pp. 52--64.

Berry, H. L. & Rickwood, D. J. 2000, 'Measuring social capital at the individual level: Personal social capital, values and psychological distress', International Journal of Mental Health Promotion, vol. 2, no. 3, pp. 35–44.

Bohle, P. & Quinlan, M. 1991, Managing Occupational Health and Safety: A Multidisciplinary Approach, Macmillan, Melbourne.

Bohle, P. & Quinlan, M. 2000, Managing Occupational Health and Safety: A Multidisciplinary Approach, 2nd edn, Macmillan, Melbourne.

Braverman, H. 1974, Labor and Monopoly Capital: Degradation of Work in the Twentieth Century, Monthly Review Press, New York.

Bryman A. 2004, Social research methods. 2nd ed. Oxford: Oxford University Press.

Bruhn, J. G. 2001, Trust and the Health of Organisations, Kluwer Academic/Plenum Publishers, New York.

Burt, R. S. 2000, 'The network structure of social capital', in Research in Organisational Behaviour, eds B. M. Straw & R. I. Sutton, Elsevier Science, Amsterdam, vol. 22, pp. 345–423.

Cairncross, F. 2001, The Death of Distance, Harvard Business School, Boston.

Caplan, R. D. 1983, 'Person-environment fit: Past, present and future', in Stress Research, ed C. L. Cooper, John Wiley & Sons Ltd, New York, pp. 35–78.

Castles, F. G. 1989, The Comparative History of Public Policy, Polity Press, Oxford.

Castles, F. G. 1999, Comparative Public Policy: Patterns of Post War Transformation, Edward Elgar, Abington.

Cohen P. 1989 'The politics of primary health care in Thailand, with special reference to non-government organisations'. In: Cohen P, Purcal J, editors. The political economy of primary health care in Southeast Asia. Canberra: The Australian National University; 1989. p.159-176.

Cohen, S. & Syme, S. L. 1985, 'Issues in the Study and Application of Social Support', in Social Support and Health, eds S. Cohen & S. L. Syme, Academic Press Inc, Orlando, pp. 3–20.

Cohen, S. & Williamson, G. M. 1991, 'Stress and Infectious Disease in Humans', Psychological Bulletin, Jan, vol. 109, no. 1, pp. 5–24.

Commission on Social Determinants of Health 2005-2008, (2011). Accessed on 15 March 2011, Available from:
http://www.who.int/social_determinants/thecommission/en/

Considine, M. 1991, The Politics of Reform: Worker's Compensation from Woodhouse to WorkCare, Deakin Series of Public Policy Administration, Melbourne, no. 1.

Considine, M. 1994, Public Policy: A Critical Approach, Macmillan, Melbourne.

Cooper, C. L. 1998, Theories of Organisational Stress, Oxford University Press, Oxford.

Cooper, C. L. & Payne, R. (eds) 1988, Causes, Coping and Consequences of Stress at Work, John Wiley & Sons Ltd, Chichester.

Cooper, C. L. 1999, 'Can we live with the changing nature of work?' Journal of Managerial Psychology, vol. 14, no. 7/8, pp. 569–572.

Cox, T. 1978, Stress, Macmillan, London.

Cox, T. & Griffiths, A. 1996, 'Assessments of Psychological Hazards', in Handbook of Work and Health Psychology, eds M. J. Schabracq, J. A. M. Winnubst & C. L. Cooper, John Wiley and Sons Ltd, Chichester, pp. 127–143.

Creighton, B. & Gunningham, N. (eds) 1985, The Industrial Relations of Occupational Health and Safety, Croom Helm, Sydney.

Creighton, B. 1993, 'Occupational Health and Safety Regulation: The Role of ILO Standards', in Work and Health, ed M. Quinlan, Macmillan, Melbourne, pp. 284–310.

Cribbs, A. & Dines, A. 1993, 'What is health?' in Health Promotion: Concepts and Practice, eds A. Cribbs & A. Dines, Blackwell, Oxford, pp. 3–19.

Crittall, J. 1995, 'Enterprise Bargaining and Occupational Health and Safety', Journal of Occupational Health Safety-Australia New Zealand, vol. 11, no. 6, pp. 587–593.

Davis, J. A., Savage, G. & Stewart, R.T. 2003, 'Organisational downsizing: a review of the literature for planning and research', Journal of Healthcare Management, vol. 48, no. 3, pp. 18–39.

Dembe, A. E. 1996, Occupation and Disease, How Social Factors Affect the Conception of Work-Related Disorders, Yale University Press, New Haven & London.

Dembe, A. E. 1999, 'Social Inequalities in Occupational Health and Health Care for Work-Related Injuries and Illness', International Journal of Law and Psychiatry, vol. 22, no. 5–6, pp. 567–579.

Denzin, N. K. 1978, The Research Act, Mc Graw Hill, New York.

Denzin, N. K. 1983, 'Interpretative Interactionism', in Beyond Method: Strategies for Social Research, ed G. Morgan, Sage Publications, Newberry Park, pp. 129–146.

Denzin, N. K. 1989, Interpretative Interactionism, Sage Publications, Newbury Park.

Denzin, N. K. & Lincoln, Y. S. (eds) 1994, Handbook of Qualitative Research, Sage Publishers, London.

Ditton, MJ 2009 The health that workers want, LAP Lambert Academic Publishing, Germany.

Ditton, MJ 2009, How social relationships influence academic health in the 'enterprise university': an insight into productivity of knowledge workers, vol 29, issue 2 pp.151-164.

Dooris, M. 2001, 'The 'Health Promoting University': a critical exploration of theory and practice', Health Education, vol. 101, no. 2, pp. 51–60.

Driscoll, T. & Mayhew, C. 1999, 'Extent and Cost of Occupational Injury and Illness', in Occupational Health and Safety in Australia: Industry, Public Sector and Small Business, eds C. Mayhew & C. Peterson, Allen & Unwin, Sydney, pp. 28–52.

Driscoll, T., Mitchell, R., Mandryk, J., Healy, S., Hendris, L. & Hull, B. 2001, 'Work- related fatalities in Australia, 1989 to 1992: An overview', J Occupational Health Safety — Aust NZ, vol. 17, no. 1, pp. 45–66.

Driskell, J. E. &. Salas, E. (eds) 1996, Stress and Human Performance, Lawrence Erlbaum, Mahwah.

Edwards, J. R. 1988, 'The Determinants and Consequences of Coping with Stress', in Causes, Coping and Consequences of Stress at Work, eds C. L. Cooper & R. Payne, John Wiley & Sons, Chichester, pp. 233–266.

Edwards, J. R., Caplan, R. D., & Van Harrison, R. 1998, 'Person-Environment Fit Theory: Conceptual Foundations, Empirical evidence and Directions for Future Research', in Theories of Organisational Stress, ed C. L. Cooper., Oxford University Press, Oxford, pp. 28–67.

Einarsen, S, Hoel, H, Zapf, and Cooper, G. 2003, 'Bullying and Emotional Abuse in the Workplace' Taylor and Francis: London.

Ellis, N. 2001, Work and Health: Management in Australia and New Zealand. Oxford University Press, Melbourne.

Emmett, T. 1999, 'Evolution of Occupational Health and Safety Policy and Programs', in Occupational Health and Safety in Australia: Industry Public Sector, and Small Business, eds C. Mayhew and C. Peterson, Allen & Unwin, Sydney, pp. 13–27.

Employment Conditions Knowledge Network (EMCONET) Final Report. (2007). Employment conditions and health inequalities. Spain. Retrieved from: http://www.who.int/social_determinants/themes/employmentconditions/en/index.html

Erez, M. &. Earley, P. C. 1993, Culture Self-identity and Work, Oxford University Press, New York.

Estes, R. 1996, Tyranny of the Bottom Line: Why Corporations make good people do bad things, Berrett-Koehler Publishers, San Francisco.

Ferrie, J. E., Shipley, M. J., Stanfeld, S.A. & Marmot, M. G. 2002, 'Effects of chronic job insecurity and change in job security on self reported health, minor psychiatric morbidity, psychological measures, and health related behaviour in British civil servants: The Whitehall 11 study (Research Report)', Journal of Epidemiology & Community Health, vol. 56, no. 6, pp. 450–456.

Filmer D, Hammer J, Pritchett L. 1997, Health policy in poor countries: weak links in the chain. Policy Research Working Paper 1874. Washington, DC: World Bank.

Foley, G. 1997, 'National Worker's Compensation-based data: Scope, coverage, benefits and uses', J Occupational Health and Safety-Aust NZ, vol. 13, no. 3, pp. 275–284.

Foley, G., Gale, J. & Gavenlock, L. 1995, 'The cost of work-related injury and disease', J Occupational Health and Safety-Aust NZ, vol. 11, no. 2, pp. 171–194.

Franks P, Clancy C, Nutting P., 1992 Sounding board: gatekeeper revisited-protecting the patient from overtreatment. N Engl J Med.327(6). p.424-429

George, J. & A. Davis 1998, States of Health: Health and Illness in Australia, Longman, Melbourne.

Giddens, A. 1979, Central Problems in Social Theory, Macmillan, London.

Gilpatrick E. 1999, Quality improvement projects in health care: problem solving in the workplace. Thousand Oaks: Sage Publications.

Grbich, C. 1996. Health in Australia Sociological Concepts and Issues, Prentice-Hall, Sydney.

Grbich, C., Mc Gartland, M. & Polgar, S. 1998, 'Regulating Workers' Compensation: the Medico-Legal evaluation of Injured Workers in Victoria', Australian Journal of Social Issues, vol. 33, no. 3, pp. 241–263.

Grbich, C. 1999, Qualitative Research in Health: An Introduction, Allen & Unwin and Sage International, St Leonards.

Gunningham, N. 1985, 'Workplace Safety and the Law', in The Industrial Relations of Occupational Health and Safety', eds B. Creighton & N. Gunningham, Croom Helm, Sydney, pp. 18–53.

Gutek, B., Repetti, R. & Silver, D. 1988, 'Nonwork Roles and Stress at Work', in Causes, Coping and Consequences of Stress at Work eds C. L. Cooper & R. Payne, John Wiley and Sons Ltd, Chichester, pp. 141–174.

Hale, A. R. & Hovden, J. 1998, 'Management and Culture: The third stage of safety. A review of approaches to organisational aspects of safety, health and environment', in Occupational Injury: Risk, Prevention and Intervention, eds A-M. Feyer, & A. Williamson, Taylor & Francis Ltd, London, pp. 129–168.

Hall, A. & Wellman, B. 1985, 'Social Networks and Social Support', in Social Support and Health, eds S. Cohen & S. L. Syme, Academic Press Inc, Orlando, pp. 23–43.

Health Promotion Glossary, (1998) Accessed on 15 March 2011, Available from: http://www.who.int/healthpromotion/about/HPG/en/index.html

Herzlich, C. & Pierret, J. 1984, Illness and Self in Society, The John Hopkins University Press, Baltimore.

Hoel, H., Rayner, C. & Cooper, C. L. 1999, 'Workplace Bullying', International Review of Industrial and Organisational Psychology, vol. 14, pp. 195–231.

Holbeche, L. 1998, Motivating People in Lean Organisations, Reed Educational and Professional Publishing Ltd, Oxford.

Holbeche, L. 1999, Aligning Human Resources and Business Strategy, Butterworth Heinemann, Oxford.

Holmes, D., Hughes, K. & Julian, R. 2003, Australian Sociology. Pearson Longman, Sydney.

Holmes, N., Triggs, T. J. & Gifford, S.M. 1997, 'Conflicting concepts of risk identification in OHS: Implications for OHS priorities', Journal of Occupational Health Safety-Aust NZ, vol. 13, no. 2, pp. 131–143.

Hopkins, A. 1993, 'Approaches to safeguarding the worker', in Work and Health: The Origins, Management and Regulation of Occupational Illness, ed M. Quinlan, Macmillan, Melbourne, pp. 170–190.

Hopkins, A. 1995, Making Safety Work, Getting Management Commitment to Occupational Health and Safety, Allen & Unwin, Sydney.

Hopkins, A. 2000, Lessons from Longford: The Esso Gas Plant Explosion, CCH Australia Ltd, North Ryde, Sydney.

Horstman, B. 1999, 'Decentralised and deregulated Australian industrial relations', Employee Relations, vol. 21, no. 3, pp. 325–341.

House, J. S. 1981, 'The Nature of Social Support', in Work stress and social support, ed J. S. House, Addison-Wiley, Reading, pp. 13–30.

House, J. S., Robbins, C. & Metzner, H. L. 1982, 'The Association of Social Relationships and Activities with Mortality: Prospective evidence from the Tecumseh Community Health Study', American Journal of Epidemiology, vol. 116, no. 1, pp.123–140.

House, J. S. & Kahn, R. L. 1985, 'Measures and Concepts of Social Support', in Social Support and Health, eds S. Cohen & S. L. Syme, Academic Press Inc, Orlando, pp. 83–104.

House, J. S., Landis, K. R. & Umberson, D. 1988, 'Social Relationships and Health', Science, July 29, vol. 241, pp. 540–545.

Howard, R. 1985, Brave New Workplace, Viking Penguin Inc, New York.

Illich, I. 1977, Limits to Medicine: Medical Nemesis: The Expropriation of Health, Penguin, Harmondsworth.

International Agency for Research on Cancer Monographs.2004 Evaluation of carcinogenic risks to humans. Betel-quid and areca-nut chewing and some areca-nut derived nitrosamines, 85 Available from: http://monographs.iarc.fr/ENG/Monographs/vol85/ volume85.pdf, [Last modified on 30/9/04]. (Accessed 19/1/07.)

International Labour Organisation, 1994, 'Constitution', The Declaration of Philadelphia, Philadelphia, USA.

International Labour Organisation, 'Strengthening Tripartism and Social Dialogue', in Information Brochure, (n.d.) [On line], Available: http://www.ilo.org/public/english/bureau/inf/brochure/index.htm, [Accessed 19 June 2004].

International Labour Organisation, Laborsta (n.d.) [Online], Available: http://laborsta.ilo.org/ [Accessed 19 June 2004].

Industry Commission, 1994, Workers' Compensation in Australia, AGPS, Canberra.

Industry Commission, 1995, Work, Health and Safety: An Inquiry into Occupational Health and Safety, AGPS, Canberra.

Jeyaratnam J. 1999, Acute pesticide poisoning: a major global health problem. World Health Statistics Quarterly. 43(3):139-144.

Jitsanguan T. Sustainable agricultural systems for small scale farmers in Thailand: implications for the environment, 2001 Taiwan: Food and Fertilizer Technology Centre; http://www.fftc.agnet.org/library/ article/eb509.html. (Accessed 3/1/06.)

Johnstone, R., (ed) 1994, Occupational Health and Safety Prosecutions in Australia. Overview and Issues, Centre for Employment and Labour Relations Law, Melbourne, Occasional Monograph Series, no. 1.

Johnstone, R. 1997, Occupational Health and Safety Law and Policy: Text and Materials, LBC Information Services, North Ryde, Sydney.

Johnstone, R. 2002, 'OHS Regulatory research: New possibilities', J Occupational Health Safety — Aust NZ, vol. 15, no. 5, pp. 3–6.

Jones, B., D. Flynn, M., & Kelloway, E. K. 1995, 'Perception of Support from the Organisation in Relation to Work Stress, in Satisfaction and Commitment', Organisational Risk Factors for Job Stress, eds S. Sauter & L. Murphy, American Psychological Association, Washington, pp. 41–52.

Jorm, A. F., Korten, A. E., Jacomb, P. A., Christensen, H., Rogers, B. & Pollitt, P. 1997, 'Mental Health Literacy: A survey of the public's ability to recognise mental disorders and their beliefs about the effectiveness of treatment', Medical Journal of Australia, vol. 166, pp. 182–186.

Kaplan, H. B. 1996, 'Themes, Lacunae, and Directions in Research on Psychological Stress', in Psychological Stress: Perspectives on Structure, Theory, Life-Course and Methods, ed H.B. Kaplan, Academic Press, San Diego, pp.369–404.

Kaplun, A. (ed) 1992. Health Promotion and Chronic Illness: Discovering a new quality of health, World Health Organization Regional Publications, European Series, Copenhagen.

Karasek, R. A. 1979, 'Job Demands, Job Decisions Latitude and Mental Strain', in Administrative Science Quarterly, reprinted in Industrial and Organisational Psychology, 1991, ed C. L. Cooper, Elgar Reference Collection, Aldershot, vol. 11, pp. 335-357.

Karasek, R. 1989, 'The political implications of psychological work redesign: A model of the psychological class structure', International Journal of Health Services, vol. 19, no. 3, pp. 481-508.

Karasek, R. 1990, 'Lower health risk with increased job control among white collar workers' Journal of Organisational Behaviour, vol. 11, pp. 171-185.

Karasek, R. & Theorell, T. 1990, Healthy Work: Stress Productivity and the Reconstruction of Working Life, Basic Books, USA.

Kemmis S, McTaggart R. 2000, Participatory action research. In: Denzin NK, Lincoln YS, editors. Handbook of qualitatie research. Thousand Oaks: Sage Publications;. p. 567-606.

Kerr, C., Morrell, S., Salked, G., Corbett, S., Taylor, R. & Webster, F. 1996, Best Estimate of the magnitude of health effects of occupational exposure to hazardous substances, AGPS, Canberra.

Kivimaki, M., Vahtera, J., Elovainio, M., Pentti, J. & Virtanen, M. 2003, 'Human costs of organisational downsizing: Comparing health trends between leavers and stayers' American Journal of Community Psychology, vol. 32, no. 1-2, pp. 57-73.

Kivimaki, M., Elovainio, M., Vahtera, J. & Ferrie, J.E. 2003, 'Organisational justice and health of employees: Prospective cohort study', Journal of Occupational and Environmental Medicine, vol. 60. no. 1, pp. 27-34.

Konradt, U., Schmook, R., & Malecke, M. 2000, 'Impacts of Telework on Individuals, Organisations, and Families-A Critical Review', in International Review of Industrial and Organisational Psychology, eds C. L. Cooper & I. T. Robertson, John Wiley & Sons, Ltd, Chichester, vol. 15, pp. 63-101.

Koopman, C., Wanat, S. F., Whitsell, S., Westrup, D. & Matano, R. 2003, 'Relationships of Alcohol Use, Stress, Avoidance Coping, and Other Factors with Mental Health in a Highly Educated Workforce', Am J Health Promotion, vol. 17, no. 4, pp. 259-268.

Kotter, J. P. 1973, 'The Psychological Contract: Managing the Joining up Process', Californian Management Review, vol. 15, no. Spring, pp. 91-99.

Kreuter, M. W. & Lezin, N. 2002, 'Social Capital Theory: Implications for Community-Based Health Promotion' in Emerging Theories in Health Promotion Practice and Research, eds R. J. DiClemente, R.A. Crosby, & M. C. Kegler, Jossey-Bass, San Francisco, pp. 228-254.

Langan-Fox, J. 1998, 'Women's Careers and Occupational Stress', in International Review of Industrial and Organisational Psychology, eds C. L. Cooper & I. T. Robertson, John Wiley & Sons, Chichester, vol. 13, pp. 273-305.

Lax, M. 2002, Occupational Medicine: Toward a Worker/Patient Empowerment Approach to Occupational Illness', International Journal of Health Services, vol. 32, no. 2, pp. 515-549.

Leigh, J. & Mayhew, C. 2002, 'Occupational risk factors in the WHO Global Burden of Disease/Comparative Risk Assessment study', J Occupational Health Safety — Aust NZ, vol. 18, no. 4, pp. 339-346.

Lincoln, Y. S. & Guba, E. G. 1985, Naturalistic Inquiry, Sage Publications, Newbury Park, CA.

Lincoln, Y.S. & Guba, E. G. 1994, 'Competing Paradigms in Qualitative Research' in Handbook of Qualitative Research, eds N. K. Denzin, & Y. S. Lincoln, pp. 105-117.

Lincoln, Y. S. & Guba, E.G. 2000, 'Paradigmatic Controversies, Contradictions, and Emerging Influences', in Handbook of Qualitative Research, eds N. K. Denzin, & Y. S. Lincoln, 2nd edn, Sage Publications, Thousand Oaks, pp. 163-188.

Lupton, D. (1995), The Imperative of Health: Public Health and the Regulated Body, Sage Publications, London.

Lynch, J., Due, P., Muntaner, C. & Davey Smith, G. 2000, 'Social capital — Is it a good investment strategy for public health?' J Epidemiology and Community Health, vol. 54, pp. 404-408.

Mandryk, J., Driscoll, T., Mazurski, E., Healy, S. & Travis, J. 2001, 'Data on occupational health and safety in Australia', J Occupational Health Safety — Aust NZ, vol. 17, no. 4, pp. 349-361.

Marginson, S. 1993, Education and Public Policy in Australia, Cambridge University Press, Cambridge.

Marginson, S. 1995, 'Markets in Higher Education: Australia', in Academic Work, ed J. Smyth, Society for Research into Higher Education & Open University Press, Buckingham, pp. 17-39.

Marginson, S. 1996, 'University Organisation in an Age of Perpetual Motion', Journal of Higher Education Policy and Management, vol. 18, no. 2, pp. 117-123.

Marginson, S. 1997, Markets in Education, Allen & Unwin, Sydney.

Marginson, S. & Considine, M. 2000, The Enterprise University: Power, Governance and Reinvention in Australia, Cambridge University Press, Cambridge.

Marmot, M. G., Shipley, M. J. & Rose, G. 1984, Inequalities in death-specific explanations of a general pattern', The Lancet, May 5, pp. 1003-1006.

Marmot, M. & Theorell, T 1988, 'Social class and cardiovascular disease: The contribution of work', International Journal of Health Services, vol. 18, no. 4, pp. 659-673.

Marmot, M. 1996, 'The social pattern of health and disease', in Health and Social Organisation, eds D. Blane, E. Brunner & R. Wilkinson, Routledge, London, pp. 42-70.

Marmot, M. & Feeney A. 1996, 'Work and Health: implications for individuals and society', in Health and Social Organisation, eds D. Blane, E. Brunner & R. Wilkinson, Routledge, London, pp. 235-254.

Marmot, M. G., Fuhrer, R. Ettner, S. L., Marks, N.F., Bumpass, L. L. & Ryff, C.D. 1998, 'Contribution of Psychological Factors to Socioeconomic Differences in Health', Millbank Quarterly, vol. 76, no. 3, pp. 403-448.

Marx, K. 1964, The Economic and Philosophic Manuscripts of 1844, International, New York,

Maslach, C. 1982, Burnout: The Cost of Caring, Prentice-Hall, New York.

Maslach, C. & Jackson, S. E. 1986, 'The Measurement of Experienced Burnout', pp. 1-14 (originally published in the Journal of Occupational Behaviour, 1981, vol. 2, pp. 99-

113) in Industrial and Organisational Psychology, 1991, ed C. L. Cooper, Algar Reference Collection, Aldershot, vol. 11, pp. 253–266.

Maslach, C. 1998, 'A Multidimensional Theory of Burnout', in Theories of Organisational Stress. ed C. L. Cooper, Oxford University Press, Oxford, pp. 68–85.

Mayhew, C., Quinlan, M. & Ferris, R. 1997, 'The Effects of SubContracting/Outsourcing on OH&S - Survey evidence from 4 Australian Industries', Safety Science, vol. 25, no. 1-3, pp. 163–178.

Mayhew, C. & Peterson, C. L. (eds) 1999a, Occupational Health and Safety in Australia: Industry, Public Sector and Small Business, Allen & Unwin, Sydney.

Mayhew, C. & Peterson, C. L. 1999b, 'Introduction: Occupational Health and Safety in Australia', in Occupational Health and Safety in Australia: Industry, Public Sector and Small Business, eds C. Mayhew & C. L. Peterson, Allen & Unwin, Sydney, pp. 1–13.

Mayhew, C. 2000, 'Funding for OHS Research in Australia', J Occupational Health Safety-Aust NZ, vol. 16, no. 3, pp. 229–232.

McCarthy, P. 1989, Developing Negotiating Skills and Behaviour, CCH Australia Limited, Sydney.

McCarthy, P., Mayhew, C., Barker, M. & Sheehan, M. 2003, 'Bullying and occupational violence in tertiary education: Risk factors, perpetrators and prevention', J Occupational Health Safety — Aust NZ, vol. 19, no. 4, pp. 319–326.

Ministry of Public Health. Standard of primary care service system (in Thai). 2001, Nakhon Ratchasima Provincial Health Office; 2001, July 18. Available from: http://www.province.moph.go.th/nakhonratchasima/ PCU/PCU_work.htm. (Accessed 8/9/06.)

Mintzberg, H. & Quinn, J. B. (eds) 1998, Readings in the Strategy Process, Prentice-Hall, Upper Saddle River.

Mintzberg, H. 1998, 'The Professional Organisation', in Readings in the Strategy Process, eds H. Mintzberg & J.B. Quinn, Prentice-Hall, Upper Saddle River, pp. 288–298.

Mrazek, P. & Haggerty, R. 1994, Reducing the Risks for Mental Disorders: Frontiers for Preventive Intervention Research, National Academy Press, Washington, DC.

Murray, R. B. 2001, 'Overview: Theories related to Human Development', in Health Promotion Strategies Through the Lifespan, eds R. B. Murray & J. P. Zentner, Prentice-Hall, Upper Saddle River, pp. 213–277.

Murray, R. B. & Zentner, J. P. (eds) 2001, Health Promotion Strategies Through the Life Span, Prentice-Hall, Upper Saddle River.

Murray, R., Zentner, J. & Samiezade-Yard, C. 2001, 'Sociocultural Influences on the Person and Family', in Health Promotion Strategies Through the Life Span, eds R. Murray & J. Zentner, Prentice-Hall, Upper Saddle River, pp. 3–71.

Naisbitt, J. & Aburdene, P. 1990, Megatrends 2000: Ten new directions for the 1990s, William Morrow and Company, New York.

National Economic and Social Development Board. Thailand's official poverty lines. 2004 Paper presented to the International Conference on Poverty Statistics, Methodology and Comparability, Manilla, Philippines 4-6 October 2004. Available from: www.nscb.gov.ph/poverty/conference/papers/7_Thai%20official%20poverty.pdf. (Accessed 12/7/2006.)

National Occupational Health and Safety Commission, 2001, Comparison of Workers' Compensation arrangements in Australia Jurisdictions, NOHSC Symposium on OHS Implications of Stress, NOHSC.

National Steering Committee on Health Promotion in the Workplace, 1989, Health at Work Information Kit, National Heart Foundation, Western Australian Division, Nedlands, WA.

Navarro, V. 1978, Medicine Under Capitalism, Prodist, New York.

Navarro, V. 2002, 'A Critique of Social Capital', International Journal of Health Sciences, vol. 32, no. 3, pp. 423-432.

Nettleton, S. 1995, The Sociology of Health and Illness, Polity Press, Cambridge.

Northwestern National Life Insurance Company. 1991, Employee Burnout: America's Newest Epidemic, Northwestern National Life Insurance Company, Minneapolis.

Norton, B.L., McLeroy, K. R., Burdine, J. N., Felix, M. R. J. & Dorsey, A. M. 2002, 'Community Capacity' in Emerging Theories in Health Promotion Practice and Research, eds R. J. DiClemente, R. A. Crosby, & M. C. Kegler, Jossey-Bass, San Francisco, pp. 194-227.

Nutbeam, D. & Harris, E. 1998, Theory in a Nutshell: A practitioner's guide to commonly used theories and models in health promotion, National Centre for Health Promotion, Sydney.

Occupational Health and Safety Act, (New South Wales), 2001.

O'Connor-Fleming, M. L. & Parker, E. 2001, Health Promotion: principles and practice in the Australian context, Allen & Unwin, Sydney.

OECD 1994, Jobs Study. Organisation for Economic Co-operation and Development, Paris.

O'Donnell, M. P. & Harris, J. S. 1994, Health Promotion in the Workplace, Delmar Publishers Inc, New York.

O'Donnell, M. P. 2001, 'Editor's Note', Am J of Health Promotion, vol. 15, no. 5, p. v.

O'Donnell, M. P. 2002, 'Why Focus on Research First?' Am J Health Promotion, vol. 17, no. 2, pp. 5-6.

Palmer, G. R. & Short, S. D. 1994, Health Care and Public Policy: An Australian Analysis, 2nd edn, Macmillan, Melbourne.

Pearse, W. & Refshauge, C. 1987, 'Worker's Health and Safety in Australia', International Journal of Health Services, vol.17, no. 4, pp. 635-650.

Per Oystein Saksvik, & Quinlan, M. 2003, 'Regulating systematic occupational health and safety management: Comparing the Norwegian and Australian experiences', Industrial Relations (Canadian), vol. 58, no.1, pp, 33-62.

Peter, R. & Siegrist, J. 1999, 'Chronic Psychological stress at Work and Cardiovascular Disease: The Role of Effort Reward Imbalance', International Journal of Law and Psychiatry, vol. 22, no. 5-6, pp. 441-449.

Petersen, A. & Lupton, D. 1996, The New Public Health: Health and Self in the Age of Risk, Allen & Unwin, St Leonards.

Petersen, D. 1990, Managing Employee Stress, Aloray Inc, New York.

Pusey, M. 1991, Economic Rationalism in Canberra: A nation building state changes its mind, Cambridge University Press, New York.

Putnam, L. L., Phillips, N. & Chapman, P. 1996, 'Metaphors of Communication and Organisation', in Handbook of Organisational Studies, eds S. T. Clegg, C. Hardy & W. R. Nord, Sage Publications, London, pp. 375-408.

Putnam, R. D. 2000, Bowling Alone: The Collapse and Revival of American Community, Simon Schuster, New York.

Quinlan, M. 1993a, 'The Industrial Relations of Occupational Health and Safety', in Work and Health, ed M. Quinlan, Macmillan, Melbourne, pp. 140-169.

Quinlan, M. 1993b, Work and Health: The Origins, Management, and Regulation of Occupational Illness, Macmillan, Melbourne.

Quinlan, M. & Mayhew, C. 1999, 'Precarious Employment and Workers' Compensation', International Journal of Law and Psychiatry, vol. 22, no. 5-6, pp. 491-520.

Quinlan, M. 2000, 'Forget Evidence: the demise of research involvement by NOHSC since 1996', Journal of Occupational Health Safety-Aust NZ, vol. 16, no. 3, pp. 213-227.

Quinlan, M. 2001/2002. 'Workplace health and safety effects of precarious employment', The Global Occupational Health Network, vol. 2, pp.1-4.

Ragin, C. C. 1991, 'The Problem of Balancing the Discourse on Cases and Variables in Comparative Social Science', in Issues and Alternatives in Comparative Social Research, eds C. C. Ragin, & E. J. Brill, Leiden, pp. 1-9.

Ransome, P. 1999, Sociology and the Future of Work: Contemporary discourses and debates, Ashgate, Aldershot.

Rawls, J. 1978, A Theory of Justice, J.W. Arrowsmith, Bristol.

Robens, Lord 1972, Report of the Committee on Safety and Health at Work 1970-1972, HMSO, London.

van Rossum, C., Shipley, M., Mheen, H., Grobbee, D. & Marmot, M. 2000, 'Employment grade differences in cause specific mortality. A 25 year follow up of civil servants from the first Whitehall study', J Epidemiology and Community Health, vol. 54, pp. 178-184.

Rousseau, D. 1995, Psychological Contracts in Organisations, Sage Publications, Thousands Oaks.

Rubery, J. 1999, 'The Fragmenting of Internal Labour Markets', in Globalisation and Labour Relations, ed P. Leisink, Edward Elgar, Cheltenham, pp. 116-137.

Russell, C. & Schofield, T 1986, Where it hurts: An Introduction to Sociology for Health Workers, Allen & Unwin, Sydney.

Russell, R. 1999, 'The Future: A Management View', in Occupational Health and Safety in Australia: Industry, Public Sector and Small Business, eds C. Mayhew & C. L. Peterson, Allen & Unwin, Sydney, pp. 86-92.

Rutter, M. 1985, 'Psychosocial resilience and protective mechanisms', American Journal of Orthopsychiatry, vol. 57, pp. 316-331.

Ryan, W. 1971, Blaming the Victim, Vintage, New York.

Sainsbury, P. 2000, 'Promoting mental health: Recent progress and problems in Australia', J Epidemiology and Community Health, vol. 54, pp. 82-83.

Sax, S. 1984, A Strife of Interests: Politics and Policies in Australian Health Services, Allen & Unwin, Sydney.

Schabracq, M. J. 2003, 'Everyday Stress and Well-being in Work and Organisations', in Handbook of Work and Health Psychology, eds M. J. Schabracq, J. A. M. Winnubst, & C. L Cooper, 2nd edn, John Wiley & Sons Ltd, Chichester, pp. 10-36.

Schabracq, M. J., Winnubst, J. A. M. & Cooper, C. L. (eds) 1996, Handbook of Work and Health Psychology, John Wiley & Sons Ltd, Chichester.

Schabracq, M. J., Winnubst, J. A. M. & Cooper, C.L. (eds) 2003, Handbook of Work and
     Health Psychology, 2nd edn, John Wiley & Sons Ltd, Chichester.

Schein, E. 1992, Organisational Culture and Leadership, Jossey Bass, San Francisco.

Scheurich, J. 1997, Research Method in the Postmodern, Falmer Press, London.

Selye, H. 1956, The Stress of Life, McGraw-Hill, New York.

Sennun P, Suwannapong N, Howteerakul N, Pacheun O. 2006,Participatory supervision
     model: building health promotion capacity among health officers and the
     community. Rural Remote Health. 6:440: Available from: http://rrh.deakin.edu.au.
     (Accessed 6/10/06.)

Short, S. 1999, 'Sociological Perspectives: Why do disadvantaged people behave badly?' in
     Perspectives in Health Inequity, eds E. Harris, P. Sainsbury & D. Nutbeam,
     Australian Centre for Health Promotion, Sydney, pp. 90–95.

Siegrist, J. 1998, 'Adverse Health Effects of Effort-Reward Imbalance at Work: Theory,
     Empirical Support and Implications for Prevention', in Theories of Organisational
     Stress, ed C. L. Cooper, Oxford University Press, Oxford, pp. 190–204.

Sigman, A. 1992, 'The state of corporate health care', Personnel Management, no. February,
     pp. 24-31.

Spillane, R. 1999, 'Australian Managers' Attitude to Mental Illness', Journal of Occupational
     Health Safety-Aust NZ, vol. 15, no. 4, pp. 359–364.

Stansfield, S., Head, J. & Marmot, M. 2000, Work related factors and ill health, The Whitehall
     11 Study, Health and Safety Executive, Norwich, pp. 1–64.

Starfield B.1994, Is primary care essential? Lancet. 344:1129-1133.

Starfield B. 1998, Primary care: balancing health needs, services and technology. New York:
     Oxford University Press.

Steenland, K., Henley, J. & Thun, M. 2002, 'All-Cause and Cause-specific Death Rates by
     Educational Status for Two Million People in the Two American Cancer Society
     Cohorts', American Journal of Epidemiology, vol. 156, no. 1, pp. 11–21.

Stiller, L., Sargaison, J. & Mitchell, T. 1998, 'Using injury data to identify industry research
     priorities', in Occupational Injury: Risk, prevention and Intervention, eds A.-M.
     Feyer & A. Williamson, Taylor & Francis, London, pp. 21–28.

Sutherland, V. J. & Cooper, C. L. 1988, 'Sources of Work Stress', in Occupational Stress:
     Issues and Developments in Research, eds J. J. Hurrell, L. R. Murphy, S. L. Sauter &
     C. L. Cooper, Taylor & Francis, New York, pp. 3–31.

Tajfel, H. 1981, Human groups and social categories, Cambridge University Press,
     Cambridge.

Terkel, S. 1972, Working: People talk about what they do all day and how they feel about
     what they do, Pantheon Books, New York.

The Nation, 2006, Bt30 health fee may be scrapped. Bangkok: The Nation. 2006 14 Oct.

Theorell, T. 1996, 'Flexibility at Work in Relation to Employee Health', Handbook of Work
     and Health Psychology, eds M. J. Schabracq, J. A. M. Winnubst & C. L. Cooper,
     John Wiley & Sons, Chichester, pp. 147–160.

Theorell, T. 1998, 'Job Characteristics in a Theoretical and Practical Health Context', in
     Theories of Organisational Stress, ed C. L. Cooper, Oxford University Press:
     Oxford, pp. 205–219.

Theorell, T. 2003, 'Commentary on: Organisational justice and health of employees: prospective cohort study', Journal of Occupational and Environmental Medicine, vol. 60, no. 1, pp. 33–34.

Tilly, C. & Tilly, C. 1998, Work under Capitalism, Westview Press, Boulder.

Turrell, G. 1995, 'Social Class and Health: A Summary of the Overseas and Australian Evidence', in Sociology of Health and Illness: Australian Readings, eds G. Lupton & J. M. Najman, Macmillan, Melbourne, pp. 113–142.

Vahtera, J., Virtanen, P., Kivimaki, M. & Pentri, J. 1999, 'Workplace as an Origin of Health Inequalities', Journal of Epidemiology and Community Health, vol. 53, no. 7, pp. 399–407.

Vahtera, J., Kivimaki, M., & Pentri, J. & Theorell, T. 2000, 'Effect of change in the psychological work environment on sickness absence: A seven year follow up of initially healthy employees', J Epidemiology and Community Health, vol. 54, pp. 488–493.

Vahtera, J., Poikolainen, K., Kivimaki, M., Ala-Muraula, L. & Pentti, J. 2002, 'Alcohol Intake and Sickness Absence: A Curvilinear Relation', American Journal of Epidemiology, vol. 156, no. 10, pp. 969–976.

Wapner, S. & Demick, J. 2000, 'Person-in-Environment Psychology: A Holistic, Developmental, Systems-Orientated Perspective', in Person-Environment Psychology, 2nd edn, eds, W. B. Walsh, K. H. Craik, & R. H. Price, Lawrence Erlbraum Associates Publishers, Mahwah, pp. 25–60.

Weimer, D. L. & Vining, A. R. (1999), Policy Analysis: Concepts and Practice, Prentice-Hall Inc, New Jersey

World Health Organization (WHO) 1946, Constitution, World Health Organization. Geneva.

WHO 1986, 'Ottawa Charter', First International Conference on Health Promotion, November1986, Ottawa, Canada.

WHO 2001, World Health Report: Mental Health: New Understanding, New Hope, World Health Organization, Geneva.

WHO,2003 Primary health care: a framework for future strategic directions, 2003 global report. Geneva: WHO.

Wibulpolprasert S, editor. Thailand health profile: 1999-2000. Bangkok: Bureau of Policy and Strategy, Ministry of Public Health; 2002.

Wibulpolprasert S, Pengpaibon P. 2003, Integrated strategies to tackle the inequitable distribution of doctors in Thailand: four decades of experience. Human Resources for Health. 1: 12: Available from: http://www.human-resources-health.com/content/1/1/12. (Accessed 11/7/06.)

Wigglesworth, E. C. 2000, 'The Current Hiatus in Occupational Injury Research in Australia', Australian and New Zealand Journal of Public Health, vol. 25, no. 1, pp. 94–97.

Wildavsky, A. 1979, Speaking Truth to Power: The Art and Craft of Policy Analysis, Transaction Publishers, New Brunswick.

Wilkinson, C. 2001, Fundamentals of Health at Work, Taylor & Francis, London.

Wilkinson, R. G. 1986, Class and Health, Tavistock Publishers, New York.

Wilkinson, R. G. 2000, 'Inequality and the social environment: A reply to Lynch et al.', Journal of Epidemiology and Community Health, vol. 54, pp. 411–413.

Williams, L. C. 1993, The Congruence of People and Organisations: Healing Dysfunction from Inside Out, Quorum Books, Westport.

Williams, S. & Cooper, L. 1999, Dangerous Waters: Strategies for Improving Well-being at Work, John Wiley, Chichester.

Winnubst, J. A. M. & Schabracq, M. J. 1996, 'Social Support, Stress and Organisations: Towards optimal matching', in Handbook of Work and Health Psychology, eds M. J. Schabracq, J. A. M. Winnubst & C. L. Cooper, John Wiley & Sons, Chichester, pp. 87–104.

WorkCover 1998, Statistical Bulletin NSW Worker's Compensation 1997–1998, WorkCover, Sydney:

WorkCover 2002a, OHS Risk Management for Supervisors and Managers, WorkCover Sydney.

Workplace Injury Management and Workers' Compensation Act, (New South Wales), 1998.

Ziglio, E. 2000, 'Repositioning health promotion', in Researching Health Promotion, eds J. Watson & S Platt, Routledge, London, pp. 23–37.

3

Craving and Indicators of Depression and Anxiety Levels in Different Time Points of Intensive Alcohol Dependence Treatment

Maja Rus-Makovec
University Psychiatric Hospital Ljubljana & School of Medicine,
University of Ljubljana
Slovenia

1. Introduction

Addiction/dependence is a chronically relapsing disorder that is characterized by a compulsion to take drugs and loss of control in limiting intake; brain stress systems can contribute to the compulsivity of drug-taking and therefore participate in the development and persistence of dependence (Koob, 2008). The concept of craving for alcohol can be recognized as a central component of the alcohol dependence syndrome together with the loss of control over and relapse to alcohol use (Anton, 1999). Gradual adaptation of brain function (neuroadaptation) to the presence of alcohol seems to be a central feature in the development of alcohol dependence (Koob & Le Moal, 2008). The neuroadaptation is not a conscious process and many alcohol dependent persons are likely to deny any craving for alcohol. Craving seems to emerge fully only when a person is prevented from access to alcohol or consciously attempts to quit alcohol use (Tiffany, 1990). Certain similarities exist between obsessive-compulsive disorder (OCD) and some aspects of craving (Anton et al., 1996) in form of recurrent and irresistible thoughts about alcohol during early recovery and during later recovery when experiencing stimulus clues or stressful states. Several scales have been developed to assess certain specific aspects of the craving phenomenon as a multidimensional and temporary phenomenon; the Obsessive Compulsive Drinking Scale (OCDS) (Anton et al., 1996) is suitable for determining the amount of craving experienced over a longer time interval (e.g. one week) and not only as a momentary urge to drink.

Concurrent depression and anxiety symptoms are among the most common problems in alcohol dependent patients: heavy drinkers with co-occurring depressive and anxiety symptoms evidence heavier alcohol use and increased risk of relapse (Hasin et al., 2007). In detoxified alcoholics, in early abstinence, overall dopaminergic neurotransmission in the ventral striatum of alcohol dependent patient is reduced. Brain studies with positron emission tomography revealed a reduction of availability and sensitivity of central dopamine D2-receptors in alcohol dependent patients, which may reflect a compensatory down-regulation after chronic alcohol intake and was associated with the subsequent relapse risk (Heinz et al., 2009). Dysfunction of dopaminergic, glutamatergic, and opioidergic neurotransmission in the brain reward system can be associated with alcohol craving. In early abstinence state of higher levels of glutamate and noradrenergic activity with lower GABA, dopaminergic and serotoninergic activity is achieved (Koob & Le Moal, 2008).

Alcohol use to relieve different affective states leads to encoded memory through the amygdale's connections with the dorsolateral prefrontal cortex and the basal ganglia; this reinforcement could support the addiction cycle. Affective stimuli, contrary to depression and anxiety, commonly associated with drinking situations can induce craving in the absence of alcohol cues, thus underlining the importance of addressing the association of (perceived) depression and anxiety with relapse (Mason et al., 2008). Craving has also been defined as the memory of the pleasant rewarding effects of drugs of abuse superimposed on a negative emotional state (Koob, 2000).

Laboratory studies of cue-elicited craving are used to evaluate the relationship between alcohol cues, behavioural responses (e.g., subjective craving ratings) and physiological responses. Regarding the association with alcohol cue reactivity most studies have found a strong relationship between craving, depressive symptoms, and anxiety symptoms among heavy drinkers (Fox et al., 2007). The study of Feldstein Ewing et al. (2010) found that cooccurring depressive and anxiety symptoms are associated with significant differential activation in key neurobiological regions in response to alcohol versus appetitive control cues with heavy drinking adults. It indicates that depressive or anxiety symptoms may increase the salience of alcohol cues, increase the perception of the positive aspect of alcohol consumption and reduce attention to the negative consequences of alcohol use (Monti et al., 2000).

Alcohol-induced depression and anxiety may be improved significantly with a sustained period of abstinence (four weeks is suggested), however they can have nature of relatively independent mental disorders' symptoms and persist beyond remission of dependent behaviour (Liappas et al., 2002). To reduce craving and improve outcome (i.e., decrease risk of relapse), treatment of depressed or anxious alcohol dependent patients therefore should address both the anxiety-depressive symptoms and the craving for alcohol, because both phenomena appear to be intertwined.

Different instruments are available to identify and/or measure the degree of alcohol dependence, among them AUDIT (Alcohol Use Disorders Identification Test) (Reinert & Allen, 2002) with summative score as a result. Instrument AUDIT detected a high prevalence of potential alcohol use disorders (Mendoza-Sassi & Beria, 2003), especially in primary care, but it lacks assessment of personality, relational and behavioural aspects. One of the very opportune measures of psychosocial implications of addictive behaviour could be subscores of SASSI instrument (The Substance Abuse Subtle Screening Inventory), declared to be the instrument, which breaks through denial (Miller et al., 1994). The SASSI outcome is conceptualised in ten subscores, allowing different dimensions of addictive behaviour to be identified. The following sub scores are obtained: FVA = face valid alcohol (acknowledged use of alcohol); FVOD = face valid other drugs (acknowledged use of other drugs); SYM = symptoms (true/false items that relate directly to substance misuse); OAT = obvious attributes (characteristics commonly associated with substance misuse); SAT = subtle attributes (basic personal style similar to substance dependent people); DEF = defensiveness (DEF tries to determine, if the client denies the existence of a substance abuse problem. DEF may or may not be related to substance abuse and that may reflect either an enduring character trait or a temporary reaction to a current situation. Low DEF score is also indicative of emotional pain.); SAM = supplemental addiction measure; FAM = family vs. controls (adult scale is based on the responses of the enabling spouses of the chemically

dependent people; the FAM measures the extent to which the client may be codependent);
COR = correctional (similarity to people with extensive legal difficulties); RAP = random
answering pattern (assesses whether or not responses are meaningful).
The treatment program at Centre for Alcohol Dependence Treatment of the University
Psychiatric Hospital Ljubljana is abstinence-based, applying a biopsychosocial paradigm
and providing integrated care for concurrent mental disorders. Treatment orientation has
been based on attempt of synthesis of different therapeutic approaches, including principles
of group, motivational enhancement therapy and (behavioural) marital and family therapy.
The intensive treatment programme has two consecutive parts: the first is inpatient
treatment, lasting about four to five weeks and the second part is provided in an every-day
outpatient setting (about six to eight weeks, depending on patients' goals and needs). The
patients' change of intensity of craving and negative affect during intensive dependence
treatment is one of the important focuses of therapists' interest. However, in reality of every
day clinical practice, patients have difficulties to identify their affect. If therapists want to
offer the personally-tailored programme of treatment, the vulnerable patients (relapse-
prone) could be better identified through understanding of interaction of craving and
negative affect (in psychiatric terms as higher levels of depression and anxiety).

1.1 The purpose of the study
In the actual research, different indicators were chosen as criterion of therapeutic effect,
among them intensity of »craving« as the most central dependent variable. The main
purpose of the actual contribution is to analyze effect of therapy from the aspect of craving
as central criterion-dependent variable, comparing three phases (time points) of therapy in
Centre for Alcohol Dependence Treatment of the University Psychiatric Hospital Ljubljana
(in the beginning; in the middle and at the end). Chosen variables, which are otherwise
treated as partial personality indicators of multiple criterion therapeutic success, are taken
into account as covariates: readiness for change in the beginning of therapy, so as perceived
levels of depression and anxiety from each of three time points of therapeutic procedure.
The intention was also to identify the structure of all just mentioned variables together.

1.2 Hypotheses
The following hypotheses were formulated:
H1: Significant differences in craving regarding different time points (therapeutic phases,
when testing occurred) exist so in the case H1a. without covariates included, as H1b. in the
case when age and degree of education, together with perceived levels of depression and
anxiety from each time point are included as covariates; H1c. no significant covariate effects
are expected.
H2: SASSI subscores, obtained at the end of therapy, H2a. mostly significantly correlate with
craving, levels of depression and anxiety from the end, but they H2b. mostly do not
correlate with levels of depression, anxiety and craving from the beginning of therapy, and,
yet H2c. SASSI subscores at the end of therapy significantly correlate with readiness for
change from the beginning of therapy.
H3: There are significant differences in chosen variables (in readiness for change, in
perceived levels of depression and anxiety, and in craving) between the groups of tested
and non tested participants, so in time point 2 (middle of the therapy), as in the time point 3

(end of therapy). Or: chosen variables from the beginning of therapy significantly discriminate between four level criterion, formed by groups of (non)tested participants in time point 2 and time point 3, on the level of at least one significant discriminate function (from three possible significant ones).

H4: Patients, who participated and who did not participate in testing in time point 3 do not differ in readiness for change and in any chosen variable from time point 1 and time point 2.

H5: Patients in different therapeutical time points significantly differ in perceived degree of own depression.

H6: Patients in different therapeutical time points significantly differ in perceived degree of their own anxiety.

Two general expectations, which could not be defined in terminology of univariate and bivariate relations, were additionally formulated:

- Age, degree of education, so as craving, perceived depression and anxiety from each of three time points form multifactorial structure; manifest variables are exclusively correlated with one of orthogonal factor.
- Craving, perceived depression and anxiety from each of three time points form multifactorial structure; manifest variables are exclusively correlated with one of orthogonal factor.

2. Method

2.1 Participants

The sample of the study included 133 patients who were consecutively recruited upon entering inpatient treatment at the Centre for Alcohol Dependence Treatment of the University Psychiatric Hospital Ljubljana (second part of the year 2009 and first part of 2010 admissions). All patients were eligible for the study. Patients were informed about study procedures and 110 patients provided written informed consent. 23 patients declined to participate. The 1st time point assessment was conducted 1week after admission to inpatient treatment (n = 110), the 2nd time point 5 weeks after admission to inpatient treatment (= beginning of day hospital) (n = 88), and the 3rd time point at the end of 10 weeks outpatient treatment (day hospital; = end of whole intensive treatment programme) (n = 73). The average age was 47.87 years (SD = 9.21). There were 27.1 % female and 72.9 % male participants. The average number of days of inpatient treatment was 35.1 (SD = 12.9) and of outpatient treatment 32.9 (SD = 20.1).

2.2 Applied instruments
2.2.1 The 1st time point

(1 week after beginning of treatment); expression "score" everywhere means summative score

- Information about demographic characteristics, medical, psychiatric, and family histories
- Questionnaires upon dependence intensity:
  - Alcohol Use Disorder Identification Test AUDIT – score (Cronbach alpha = 0.88; ten items with answering scale from 0 to 4) (Reinert & Allen, 2002).
  - The Substance Abuse Subtle Screening Inventory SASSI – 10 sub scores (Miller et al., 1994).

- Obsessive Compulsive Drinking Scale – score (Cronbach alpha =0.90; scale with 14 questions with mostly five points answering scale from 0 to 4, only one item from 1 to 5) (Anton et al., 1995).
- The Stages of Change Readiness and Treatment Eagerness Scale SOCRATES score (19 items of Likert type five points answering scale, Cronbach alpha = 0.95; Cronbach alphas of subscores Recognition = 0.87, Ambivalence = 0.78, Taking Steps = 0.92; correlations total score and subscores, all p < 0.001: Recognition 0.93, Ambivalence 0.89, Taking Steps 0.93) (Miller & Tonigan, 1996).
- State Anxiety Inventory – score (Cronbach alpha =0.93); twenty items with four points answering scale (Spielberger et al., 1983).
- Zung Self-Rating Depression Scale – score (Cronbach alpha =0.86; all together 20 items with four points answering scale (Zung, 1965).
- Family climate questionnaire – score (Cronbach alpha = 0.90;); originally constructed by Rus-Makovec M. et collaborators as summative scale/semantic differential, 15 bipolar continuums of semantic differential, with 7 – point bipolar answering scale, constructed according to the demands for summative ratings.

2.2.2 The 2nd time point
(5 weeks after beginning of treatment)
- More complex autoanamnestic information
- Questionnaire upon dependence intensity:
    - Obsessive Compulsive Drinking Scale – score (Cronbach alpha =0.94)
- State Anxiety Inventory – score (Cronbach alpha =0.96)
- Trait Anxiety Inventory – score (Cronbach alpha = 0.94)
- Zung Self-Rating Depression Scale – score (Cronbach alpha =0.91)
- Life events in last 12 months
- The Mini-International Neuropsychiatric Interview (M.I.N.I.)(Sheehan et al., 1998).

2.2.3 The 3rd time point
(at the end of whole intensive treatment – about 10 weeks after beginning of treatment)
- Evaluation of different components of the programme, different self evaluations
- Questionnaires upon dependence intensity:
    - The Substance Abuse Subtle Screening Inventory SASSI
    - Obsessive Compulsive Drinking Scale– score (Cronbach alpha =0.89)
- State Anxiety Inventory – score (Cronbach alpha = 0.94)
- Zung Self-Rating Depression Scale – score (Cronbach alpha = 0.89)
- Family climate questionnaire – score (Cronbach alpha = 0.91).

The whole research is designed as one–group quasi–experimental approach, with no simultaneously control such as group neither in therapeutic nor in after care period. Anyway, comparison with certain quasi-control groups, comparing particular chosen variables is possible, but not included into present report. Univariate, bivariate and multivariate statistical analyses were executed, when parametric approaches permitted. There was a problem connecting decisions for within–subjects (repeated measures) and between-subjects approach (independent groups). Only a small segment of the whole project results is shown here.

Ethical approval was provided by the Ethical commission of Health Ministry of Slovenia.

3. Results

3.1 Results of verification of hypothesis H1 - H1a

"Cravings" (Obsessive Compulsive Drinking Scale – score) in each of three time points were compared and tests of within – subject's effects without any covariate were applied. Zero risk level of differences between the periods of therapy showed highly significant differences between the cravings (F (2, 114) = 44.29, p = 0.00, part. η^2 = 0.44). Repeated measure approach embraced all together n = 58 patients, because several dozens of the declined to be tested in each of three periods/time points. The results show, approaching to the end of therapy, progressively lower and lower level of craving (Table 1).

	M	SD	N
Craving 1	24.77	10.29	58
Craving 2	15.93	12.14	58
Craving 3	10.31	8.88	58

Note:
Craving i (i = 1, 2, 3) = Obsessive Compulsive Drinking Scale – score (three time points, the first one = 1, the second one = 2, the third one = 3).

Table 1. Descriptive statistics for cravings in three time points – repeated measures approach without covariates.

3.2 Results of verification of hypothesis H1b and H1c

In the next step, nine covariates were included into the already existing repeated measures (within – subjects) design. Almost all covariate effects were found as non – significant, except two of them: years of education (F $_{educ}$ (2, 68) = 3.01, p = 0.056) and depression 1 (in the beginning/ the first time point (F $_{depr1}$ (2, 68) = 5.8, p = 0.005). When covariates included, the differences between the "cravings" were not found significant (F $_{factor1}$ (2, 68) = 1.22, p = 0.30). The function of mentioned depression is the complex one. It does not belong to the same factor (factor analysis) as "craving 3", but it significantly contributes to the understanding of the within – subjects differences between the time points. Other results were as follows: F $_{SOCRATES}$ (2, 68) = 0.26, p = 0.77; F $_{anks1}$ (2, 68) = 1.16, p = 0.32; F $_{depr2}$ (2, 68) = 0.45, p = 0.64; F $_{anks2}$ (2, 68) = 0,54, p = 0.59; F $_{depr3}$ (2, 68) = 1.34, p = 0.27; F $_{anks3}$ (2, 68) = 0.62, p = 0.54 ; F $_{age}$ (2, 68) = 2.00, p = 0.14.

	M	SD	N
Craving 1	23.93	10.60	44
Craving 2	14.02	11.35	44
Craving 3	10.27	9.15	44

Note:
Craving i (i = 1, 2, 3) = Obsessive Compulsive Drinking Scale – score (three time points, the first one = 1, the second one = 2, the third one = 3).
Covariates: depression and anxiety in each of three time points, readiness for change, age and years of education.

Table 2. Descriptive statistics for cravings in three time points – repeated measures approach with nine covariates.

I also wanted to know, what happens, when "only" seven covariates, without "age" and "years of education" are included (covariates: depression and anxiety in each of three time

Craving and Indicators of Depression and Anxiety Levels in Different Time Points of Intensive Alcohol
Dependence Treatment

69

points and readiness for change - seven covariates). Again, only the depression, as perceived in the beginning of therapy (F $_{depr1}$ (2, 92) = 7.06, p = 0.00), had a significant covariate effect on »craving«, and »within – subjects« effect was highly non – significant (F factor1 (2, 92) = 0.23, p =0.79). Covariate effects of »depressions« and »anxieties«, as perceived in other time points, were found as follows: F $_{depr1}$ (2, 92) = 7.06, p = 0.00; F $_{anxi1}$ (2, 92) = 0.43, p = 0.65; F $_{depr2}$ (2, 19) = 0.19, p = 0.89; F $_{anxi2}$ (2, 92) = 0.90, p = 0. 41; F $_{depr 3}$ (2, 92) = 0.82, p =0.44; F $_{anxi3}$ (2, 92) = 0.34, p = 0.71. Highly non – significant was also the covariate effect of the readiness for the change (SOCRATES): F $_{SOCRATES}$ (2, 92) =0.22, p =0.80.

	M	SD	n
Craving 1	24.62	10.23	54
Craving 2	15.98	12.07	54
Craving 3	10.25	8.78	54

Note:
Craving i (i = 1, 2, 3) = Obsessive Compulsive Drinking Scale – score (three time points, the first one = 1, the second one = 2, the third one = 3).
Covariates: depression and anxiety in each of three time points and readiness for change.

Table 3. Descriptive statistics for cravings in three time points – repeated measures approach with seven covariates.

3.3 Results of verification of hypothesis H2a and H2c

SASSI subscores at the end of treatment	Craving 1	SOCRATES	Depression 1	Anxiety 1
FVA	0.231	0.016	0.165	0.170
FVOD	0.009	0.004	0.218	0.204
SYM	0.236	-0.129	0.239	0.162
OAT	0.128	-0.092	0.185	0.196
SAT	0.236	0.000	0.094	0.230
DEF	-0.294*	-0.086	-0.327**	-0.265*
SAM	-0.186	-0.081	-0.099	0.061
FAM	-0.100	0.167	-0.152	-0.182
COR	0.304*	-0.044	0.315*	0.244

Note:
number of participants 65 = > n > = 64
SASSI subscores: FVA = face valid alcohol; FVOD = face valid other drugs; SYM = symptoms; OAT = obvious attributes; SAT = subtle attributes; DEF = defensiveness; SAM = supplemental addiction measure; FAM = family vs. controls; COR = correctional
Craving 1 = Obsessive Compulsive Drinking Scale – score, the first time point
Depression 1 = Zung Self-Rating Depression Scale – score, the first time point
Anxiety 1= State Anxiety Inventory – score, the first time point
SOCRATES = readiness for change in the beginning of therapy.

Table 4. Spearman coefficients of rank correlations between subscores of SASSI at the end of therapy and chosen variables from the beginning of therapy.
*, p < 0.05; **, p < 0.01

3.4 Results of verification of hypothesis H2b and H2c

SASSI subscores at the end of treatment	Craving 3	SOCRATES	Depression 3	Anxiety 3
FVA	0.408**	0.016	0.204	0.211
FVOD	-0.166	0.004	0.108	0.244*
SYM	0.219	-0.129	0.248*	0.175
OAT	0.268*	-0.092	0.405**	0.279*
SAT	-0.014	0.000	-0.039	0.214
DEF	-0.366**	-0.086	-0.550**	-0.560**
SAM	0.276*	-0.081	0.128	-0.005
FAM	-0.084	0.167	-0.261*	-0.404**
COR	0.264*	-0.044	0.410**	0.240

Note:

number of participants $65 = > n > = 64$

SASSI subscores: FVA = face valid alcohol; FVOD = face valid other drugs; SYM = symptoms; OAT = obvious attributes; SAT = subtle attributes; DEF = defensiveness; SAM = supplemental addiction measure; FAM = family vs. controls; COR = correctional

Craving 3 = Obsessive Compulsive Drinking Scale – score, the third time point

Depression 3 = Zung Self-Rating Depression Scale – score, the third time point

Anxiety 3 = State Anxiety Inventory – score, the third time point

SOCRATES = readiness for change in the beginning of therapy.

Table 5. Spearman coefficients of rank correlations between subscores of SASSI at the end of therapy and chosen variables from the end of therapy, *, $p < 0.05$; **, $p < 0.01$

I was also interested into the question, how do SASSI subscores at the end of therapy correlate with the craving, depression, readiness for change and anxiety, so from the beginning, as from the end of therapy. When four chosen variables from the beginning of therapy were taken into account, craving 1 correlated significantly ($p < 0.05$) with DEF and COR and almost significantly with SYM and SAT. Craving 3 correlated significantly with FVA, OAT, DEF, SAM and COR. It seems that correlations with DEF and COR are stable: correlations between craving and FVA, OAT and SAM appear as new significant ones at the end of therapy. Lower defensiveness at the end of the intensive treatment is significantly correlated with higher levels of craving and more intense negative affective states in beginning of treatment (and vice versa); the same trend can be seen with craving and negative affect at the end of treatment.

No significant correlations were found between SASSI subscores on one side and readiness for change on another side. They were found neither in the beginning, nor at the end of therapy.

DEF and COR correlated significantly with the depression, as perceived so in the beginning, as at the end of therapy. At the end, significant correlations were found also for SYM, OAT and FAM.

Anxiety, as perceived in the beginning, correlated significantly ($p < 0.05$) with the DEF and almost significantly with the COR. At the end of therapy, significant correlations with FAM and OAT appeared.

3.5 Results of verification of hypothesis H3

There was a variation in testing participation in each time point; that's why I decided to compare those, who participated and who did not participate testing in the second and in the third time point (= end of therapy). In such a case, the only possible comparison is comparison in variables from previous time points, in which they had participated. Mentioned comparisons are important also for the evaluation of the repeated measures design. If there are not significant differences in particular relevant previous variable between the participants and non – participants in particular time point of testing, also the validity of within – subjects (repeated measures) design is greater, although reduced number of people is taken into account.

The following proportions of (non) participants in the second and in the third time point could be identified:

M2 = proportions of participants, who: 1 = participated in the second time point, 2 = did not participate in the second time point.

M3 = proportions of participants, who: 1 = participated in the third time point, 2 = did not participate in the third time point.

Four groups with regard to participation	variable	M	SD
1 n = 51	SOCRATES	81.19	12.26
	Craving 1	24.97	10.04
	Depression 1	40.59	9.84
	Anxiety 1	38.40	12.99
2 n = 28	SOCRATES	80.81	8.53
	Craving 1	25.25	8.80
	Depression 1	40.23	8.54
	Anxiety 1	40.07	13.06
3 n = 18	SOCRATES	79.77	18.20
	Craving 1	19.77	8.86
	Depression 1	38.28	7.34
	Anxiety 1	36.88	10.94
4 n = 6	SOCRATES	88.16	6.24
	Craving 1	26.83	7.54
	Depression 1	39.33	9.89
	Anxiety 1	35.33	12.09
Total n= 103	SOCRATES	81.25	12.42
	Craving 1	24.21	9.48
	Depression 1	39.99	8.98

Note:
Craving 1 = Obsessive Compulsive Drinking Scale – score, the first time point
Depression 1 = Zung Self-Rating Depression Scale – score, the first time point
Anxiety 1 = State Anxiety Inventory – score, the first time point
SOCRATES = readiness for change in the beginning of therapy.

Table 6. Descriptive statistics for chosen variables from the beginning of therapy for four groups: groups of (non)participants in the second and in the third time point with chose

Four groups could be formed as criterion for discriminant analysis, if M2 and M3 are crossed (1 = participated in the second and in the third (n = 51); 2 = participated in the second, not in the third (n = 28); 3 = did not participate in the second, but participated in the third time point (n = 18); 4 = participated neither in the second, nor in the third time point (n = 6)). Chosen variables from the beginning of therapy were treated as predictors.

Test of Function(s)		Wilks' Lambda	Chi-square	df	Sig.
	1 through 3	0.922	7.557	12	0.819
Dimension	2 through 3	0.974	2.409	6	0.879
	3	0.995	0.462	2	0.794

Table 7. Wilks' Lambda for three discriminant functions
Box's M, F approx = 1.45, p = 0.054

Otherwise, the demand for homogeneity of covariance's was just satisfied (Box's M, F approx = 1.45, p = 0.054). Wilks' test of equality of group means, otherwise included as option of multivariate discriminant test, showed no significant differences in any of chosen variables from the beginning of therapy, when four groups were compared (look Table 11, please). Also no one of three discriminant function was found as significant: no Wilks Lambda was significant (look, please Table 12) and further analysis in the sense of discriminant analysis was not any more relevant (for example, the interpretation of structure matrix, where the degree of correlation between the (significant) discriminant function and particular predictor (chosen variables from the beginning of therapy) explain relative importance of particular predictor for the discrimination between the levels of variation of criterion (in "our" case four groups of (non)participants) and four possible centroids for each of eventually three possible significant discriminant functions.

3.6 Results of verification of hypothesis H4

Variables	M3	n	M	SD	t	df	p
Craving 2	1	53	15.60	11.97	-0.207	80	0.836
	2	29	16.17	11.69			
SOCRATES	1	66	80.69	13.93	0.079	98	0.937
	2	34	80.47	12.94			
Depression 1	1	69	40.33	9.15	0.310	103	0.757
	2	36	39.76	8.71			
Anxiety 1	1	68	38.41	12.31	-0.173	102	0.863
	2	36	38.86	13.03			
Craving 1	1	69	23.18	10.56	-1.251	101	0.214
	2	34	25.79	8.49			
Depression 2	1	53	36.79	8.36	0.224	80	0.823
	2	29	36.37	7.18			
Anxiety 2	1	55	36.58	12.29	-0.482	82	0.631
	2	29	38.00	13.76			

Note:
M3 = 1 = those, who participate testing in the third time point; M3 = 2 = those, who did not participate testing at the end of therapy:

Craving 1 = Obsessive Compulsive Drinking Scale – score in the first time point
Depression 1 = Zung Self-Rating Depression Scale – score in the first time point
Anxiety 1= State Anxiety Inventory – score in the first time point
Craving 2 = Obsessive Compulsive Drinking Scale – score in the second time point
Depression 2 = Zung Self-Rating Depression Scale – score in the second time point
Anxiety 2 = State Anxiety Inventory – score in the second time point
SOCRATES = readiness for change in the beginning of therapy.

Table 8. T – tests of difference in chosen variables regarding two groups of participants: those, who participated vs. those, who did not participate testing at the end of therapy

When those, who did not participate the testing at the end of therapy, were compared with those, who had passed the testing, no significant difference for any of treated variable (readiness, craving, depression, anxiety – so from the first, as from the second time point) was found. The results contribute to belief that "missing persons" at the end of therapy do not change the mainstream therapeutic effects.

3.7 Results of verification of hypothesis H5

	M	SD	n
Depression 1	40.39	9.58	56
Depression 2	35.55	7.75	56
Depression 3	35.53	8.44	56

Note:
Depression i (i = 1, 2, 3) = Zung Self-Rating Depression Scale – score
(three time points, the first one = 1, the second one = 2, the third one = 3).

Table 9. Descriptive statistics for perceived depression in three time points – repeated measures approach

Within subjects approach showed significant differences in perceived depression in the beginning compared to perceived depression in the middle and at the end of therapy (F (2, 110) = 15.93, p = 0.00). No significant difference appears between time point 2 and time point 3 (between middle and the end of therapy).

3.8 Results of verification of hypothesis H6

	M	SD	n
Anxiety 1	39.41	13.56	56
Anxiety 2	35.58	12.95	56
Anxiety 3	35.44	12.00	56

Note:
Anxiety i (1 = 1, 2, 3) = State Anxiety Inventory – score
(three time points, the first one = 1, the second one = 2, the third one = 3).

Table 10. Descriptive statistics for own perceived anxiety in three time points – repeated measures approach

Within subjects approach showed significant differences in perceived anxiety in the beginning compared to perceived anxiety in the middle and at the end of therapy (F (2, 110)

= 5.02, p = 0.01). No significant difference appears between time point 2 and time point 3 (between middle and the end of therapy).

3.9 Factor solutions for different set of variables
3.9.1 Factor analysis for 9 variables

Component		Initial Eigenvalues			Extraction Sums of Squared Loadings		
		Total	% of Variance	Cumulative %	Total	% of Variance	Cumulative %
dimension	1	4.412	49.018	49.018	4.412	49.018	49.018
	2	1.651	18.347	67.365	1.651	18.347	67.365
	3	0.952	10.577	77.942	0.952	10.577	77.942
	4	0.531	5.895	83.838			

Note:
Table is reduced to number of factors which sufficiently show, how many factors have the eigenvalue > = 1
(Kaiser's criterion), df = 36.

Table 11. Factor analysis for 9 variables: eigenvalues and correspondent percents of explained variance

Taking formalistically into account Kaiser's criterion, two factorial model would be taken into account, with about 67 % of explained variance. Anyway, also three factorial, explaining almost 78 % of the whole variance, could be taken into account (the eigenvalue of the third factor is 0.95 and the first three factors, according to their Kaiser values, distinctively enough separate from other factors).

Variables	Component	
	1	2
Craving 1	-0.050	0.859
Craving 2	0.123	0.836
Craving 3	0.129	0.450
Depression 1	0.576	0.513
Depression 2	0.896	0.132
Depression 3	0.873	0.187
Anxiety 1	0.774	0.036
Anxiety 2	0.872	0.214
Anxiety 3	0.876	0.012

Note:
Craving i (i = 1, 2, 3) = Obsessive Compulsive Drinking Scale – score
(three time points, the first one = 1, the second one = 2, the third one = 3)
Depression i (i = 1, 2, 3) = Zung Self-Rating Depression Scale – score
(three time points, the first one = 1, the second one = 2, the third one = 3)
Anxiety i (I = 1, 2, 3) = State Anxiety Inventory – score
(three time points, the first one = 1, the second one = 2, the third one = 3.

Table 12. Rotated varimax matrix for nine studied variables - two factorial solution

Craving and Indicators of Depression and Anxiety Levels in Different Time Points of Intensive Alcohol
Dependence Treatment

75

Variables	Component		
	1	2	3
Craving 1	-0.036	**0.863**	0.117
Craving 2	0.136	**0.823**	0.162
Craving 3	0.125	0.181	**0.943**
Depression 1	**0.589**	**0.603**	-0.247
Depression 2	**0.898**	0.098	0.088
Depression 3	**0.875**	0.158	0.081
Anxiety 1	**0.776**	0.052	-0.085
Anxiety 2	**0.874**	0.164	0.153
Anxiety 3	**0.874**	-0.032	0.103

Note:
Craving i (i = 1, 2, 3) = Obsessive Compulsive Drinking Scale – score
(three time points, the first one = 1, the second one = 2, the third one = 3)
Depression i (i = 1, 2, 3) = Zung Self-Rating Depression Scale – score
(three time points, the first one = 1, the second one = 2, the third one = 3)
Anxiety i (I = 1, 2, 3) = State Anxiety Inventory – score
(three time points, the first one = 1, the second one = 2, the third one = 3.

Table 13. Rotated component matrix for nine studied variables – three factorial solution

Factor saturation shows the same trends so for two-, as for three-factorial models. "Craving 3" is either correlated with no factor (two-factorial), or it exclusively relatively highly correlates with the third factor (three factorial solutions).

3.9.2 Factor analysis for 12 variables

Component		Initial Eigenvalues			Extraction Sums of Squared Loadings		
		Total	% of Variance	Cumulative %	Total	% of Variance	Cumulative %
dimension	1	4.783	39.86	39.86	4.78	39.86	39.86
	2	1.812	15.10	54.96	1.81	15.10	54.96
	3	1.514	12.61	67.57	1.51	12.61	67.57
	4	0.876	7.30	74.87			

Note:
Table is reduced to number of factors which sufficiently show how many factors have the eigenvalue > = 1
(Kaiser's criterion).

Table 14. Factor analysis for 12 variables: eigenvalues and correspondent percents of explained variance

Factor analysis for 12 variables resulted in three factorial solution, all three factors together explaining almost 68 % of total variance. Relatively the greatest percent of explained variance corresponds, of course, with the first factor (almost 40 %).

Varimax orthogonal rotation was applied, resulting in rotated matrix with three recognizable and relatively exclusive factors. According to the correlations between particular factor and each of 12 manifest variables, the factors could be interpreted as follows: the first factor, highly correlating with depression and anxiety, regardless the time

Variables	Component		
	1	2	3
Age	-0.063	-0.057	**0.669**
Years of education	-0.025	0.211	**0.829**
Craving 1	0.121	**0.822**	0.050
SOCRATES	-0.136	**0.688**	0.216
Craving 2	0.198	**0.663**	-0.470
Craving 3	0.233	0.432	-0.407
Depression 1	**0.800**	0.264	0.104
Anxiety 1	**0.733**	-0.083	-0.169
Depression 2	**0.875**	0.145	-0.185
Anxiety 2	**0.901**	0.151	-0.148
Depression 3	**0.895**	0.044	-0.074
Anxiety 3	**0.894**	-0.085	0.000

Note:
Craving i (i = 1, 2, 3) = Obsessive Compulsive Drinking Scale – score
(three time points, the first one = 1, the second one = 2, the third one = 3)
Depression i (i = 1, 2, 3) = Zung Self-Rating Depression Scale – score
(three time points, the first one = 1, the second one = 2, the third one = 3)
Anxiety i (I = 1, 2, 3) = State Anxiety Inventory – score
(three time points, the first one = 1, the second one = 2, the third one = 3)
SOCRATES = readiness for change in the beginning of therapy

Table 15. Rotated matrix – varimax rotation for 12 manifest variables

point of their appearance, could be labelled as »affect« factor. – The second factor exclusively highly correlates with "craving" in the beginning and in the middle (the second time point), but also with the readiness for change in the beginning of therapy; this combination could be called as before final craving & initial readiness for improvement. Finally, the third factor is a demographic one, containing age and years of education.
Final »craving« quite moderately correlates so with the second (positively), as with the third Factor (negatively) but craving 3 correlate expressively with no one of three orthogonal factors.

4. Discussion

Results show, that significant differences in craving regarding different time points (therapeutic phases, when testing occurred) exist in the case H1a. without covariates included; this hypothesis is completely confirmed, but hypothesis H1b. is refused. When age and degree of education, together with perceived anxiety and depression from each time point are included as covariates, the within subjects differences between the cravings are not any more significant. Refused is also hypothesis H 1c. (no significant covariate effects are expected), because quite significant covariate effect of perceived depression was found and almost significant effect of "years of education".
We can say, although it sounds a little bit strange, that H2a and H2b are mostly accepted (H2: SASSI subscores, obtained at the end of therapy, H2a. mostly significantly correlate with craving, depression and anxiety from the end, but they H2b. mostly do not correlate with anxiety, depression and craving from the beginning of therapy), but hypothesis H2 c is surprisingly refused, because no one significant correlation between SASSI subscores at the end of therapy and beginning readiness for change was found.

Results show that H3 (chosen variables from the beginning of therapy significantly discriminate between four level criterion, formed by groups of (non)tested participants in time point 2 and time point 3, on the level of at least one significant discriminate function (from three possible significant ones) is refused.

Also the H4 was refused (H4: Patients, who participated and who did not participate in testing in time point 3 differ in readiness for change and in any chosen variable from time point 1 and time point 2).

As expected, the alternative hypotheses H5 & H6 were confirmed. Anyway, it's worth repeating again, that significant difference (p < 0.05) was found only between time point 1 on one side and time point 2 on other side. It means that perceived depression and anxiety were significantly diminished already in the time point 2 (in the middle of therapy) and that they did not significantly change up to the end of therapy.

We can say that age, degree of education, so as craving, perceived depression and anxiety from each of three time points form multifactorial structure, "where" manifest variables are exclusively correlated with one of orthogonal factor. Factor analysis resulted in three factorial orthogonal structure with factors representing anxiety and depression (factor1), craving1, craving 2 and beginning readiness for change (factor 2) and age and years of education as factor 3. Craving 3 correlated expressively with no one of three orthogonal factors, but more strongly with factor 2 and factor 3 than with factor 1.

Factor solutions showed some interesting differences when different sets of variables were factorized. Results of factorization of 12 variables were already previously mentioned. When nine variables (perceived depression and anxiety) were factorized, so two-factorial, as three factorial model shows very similar trends; factually, the only difference between them is connected with "craving 3" (phenomenon of craving at the end of therapy). In two factorial models, craving factually "belongs" to no factor, but in three factorial models it's expressively the independent one, representing the third factor. Otherwise, so two-, as three – factorial model confirm the fact, that perceived depression in the beginning of therapy ("depression 1") "belongs" so to factor 1, as to factor 2; it means that it independently belongs so to the first (expressing anxieties and depressions in three therapeutic periods) as to the second factor (correlating with craving1 and craving 2, but not also with the craving 3).

It seems, also after a vast survey of relevant literature that analyses of relations between craving and perceived depression/anxiety are relatively very rare, especially in the framework of longitudinal, time points approach. Yet some of the studies addressed perceived depression/anxiety as a significant predictor of alcohol relapse, as well as the relation between perceived depression/anxiety and drinking, which is strongly mediated by alcohol craving (Conner et al., 2009). The craving module of the combined behavioural intervention (Witkiewitz et al., 2011) and Mindfulness-based relapse prevention were found to weaken the relation between perceived depression/anxiety and heavy drinking by fostering greater decreases in craving during treatment (Witkiewitz & Bowen, 2010). In a study of examination the course of affective symptoms and cravings for alcohol use during the initial 25 days of residential treatment addicted to alcohol, 17 subjects reported elevated cravings during the entire treatment stay, 37 subjects reported initially elevated but a slight improvement in craving, and 41 subjects reported relatively low craving from the time of admission to the end of residential treatment. Alcohol craving class was associated with perceived depression/anxiety but not with affects, being contrary to depression and anxiety; results suggested that non-cue induced alcohol craving may define a subtype of alcohol dependence that is less responsive to treatment and may explain heterogeneity in treatment outcomes (Oslin et al., 2009).

The present study's outcomes reflect neurobiological interrelation between craving and perceived depression/anxiety (described in the introductory part). The findings showed positive outcome of researched indicators of therapy success, which can be generalised to whole sample; it seems that "missing persons" at the end of therapy do not change the mainstream therapeutic effects. However, the main advantage of the study is in providing important evidence-based support to dynamics of patients' multilevel mental vulneralibility/health change in treatment process. Craving intensity diminished significantly from the beginning to very end of whole intensive treatment. Comparing to the beginning of therapy, craving in any further time point was found as significantly lower. The second time point is at the beginning of outpatient part of treatment, with exposition to environmental alcoholic and non-alcoholic cues of »real life«. Patients, involved in intensive mixture of spectrum of psychotherapy interventions and pharmacotherapy, together with abstinence, are reliably prepared for better beginner coping with higher levels of depression, anxiety and craving. On the other hand, just mentioned levels of depression and anxiety are significantly diminished (together with craving) in the first part of intensive treatment (inpatient/residential part). In times of economic crisis, inpatient treatments of dependence maybe won't be encouraged, but in-patient treatment of alcohol dependence at the beginning of the treatment process obviously can provide context for efficient sustaining at least several weeks of abstinence, allowing craving and affect issues to be addressed efficiently.

One of the expected goals for the patients in treatment of dependence from the side of the therapists is that patients diminish their denial. Correlations between SASSI subscores, craving, levels of depression and anxiety showed particular similar trend so in the beginning, as at the end of therapy. Significant correlations (higher at the end than in the beginning) between craving, levels of depression and anxiety on one side with SASSI subscore DEF on the other side appeared. Participants, who experienced more intense craving and higher levels of depression/anxiety, showed less defensiveness so in the beginning, as at the end of therapy, when the mentioned trend is much more expressed. It can be interpreted, that more vulnerable patients show less defensiveness significantly, but less expressively in the beginning and significantly, but more expressively at the end of treatment. Or patients, who do not tend to be alexitimic, show less denial with regard to their affect and craving. It is concordant with psychodynamic explanation that only patients, who are progressing in treatment and have developed good working alliance, can experience, identify and tolerate higher levels of depression and anxiety - and develop more self-defensive behaviour (Weegmann, 2002).

Weakness of the research is in the fact of missing values, which specially appear in the second and in the third (the end of therapy) time point. This deficiency has somehow tried to be controlled with comparison, in chosen target variables, between participants and non-participants in particular time point. No significant difference was found in any variable (readiness for change, perceived depression, anxiety, and craving) from the beginning of therapy. It means that those, who in some later phase did not participate testing had been not, in the beginning of therapy, differently oriented connecting some basic relevant variables of the research. Not the systematic, but random factors seem to be more relevant reason of their absence in some periods (time points) of testing.

The next weakness of the design is the absence of the adequate control group; that's why the whole design is the one – group quasi experimental one; however, there is a possibility to establish some other groups as quasi control ones. In the same time, this opportunity is, in the same time, the potential (future) advantage of the research: the same set of instruments could be applied on approximately equalized group, what would make some comparisons possible and relevant. Finally, an additional instrument, measuring some personality structure characteristics, is also supposed to be added in the future, including also some other feelings and emotions of patients in treatment (not only levels of depression and anxiety).

5. Conclusion

Quite important characteristic of the research is the institutional framework of its realization and application. This framework is the Centre for Alcohol Dependence Treatment of the University Psychiatric Hospital Ljubljana, where it is possible to take results of the study into account in applied work and longitudinally follow up. This situation also gives the opportunities for additional specification of evidence based treatment at the centre.
Projects for the future: the same group of ex- patients will be followed also in the future and the new time points will be added.

6. Acknowledgment

I would like to thank Vida Tomsic and Matjaz Mohar for their technical support.

7. References

Anton, F.R., Moak, H.D. & Latham, P. (1995). The Obsessive Compulsive Drinking Scale: A Self-Rated Instrument for the Quantification of Thoughts about Alcohol and Drinking Behavior, *Alcoholism: Clinical and Experimental Research*, Vol.19, No1, pp. 92–99, ISSN 0145-6008

Anton, R.F., Moak, D.H. & Latham, P.K. (1996). The Obsessive Compulsive Drinking Scale (OCDS): A new method of assessing outcome in alcoholism treatment studies, *Archives of General Psychiatry*, No.53, pp. 225-231, ISSN 0003990X

Anton, F.R. (1999). What is craving? *Alcohol Res Health*, Vol.23, No3, pp. 165-73, ISSN 0090-838X

Conner, K.R., Pinquart, M. & Gamble, S.A. (2009). Meta-analysis of depression and substance use among individuals with alcohol use disorders, *J Subst Abuse Treat*, Vol.37, No.2, pp. 27-137, ISSN 0740-5472

Feldstein Ewing, W.S., Filbey, M.F., Chandler, D.L. & Hutchison, K.E. (2010). Exploring the relationship Between Depressive and Anxiety Symptoms and neural response to Alcohol Cues, *Alcohol Clin Exp Res*, Vol.34, No.3, pp. 396-403, ISSN 1530-0277

Fox, H.C., Bergquist, K.L., Hong, K.I. & Sinha, R. (2007). Stress-induced and alcohol cue-indiced craving in recently abstinent alcohol dependent individuals. *Alcohol Clin Exp Res*, No.31, pp.395-403, ISSN 1530-0277

Hasin, D.S., Stinson, F.S., Ogburn, E. & Grant, B.F. (2007). Prevalence, correlates, disability, and comorbidity of DSM-IV alcohol abuse and dependence in the United States: results from the National Epidemiologic Survey on Alcohol and Related Conditions, *Arch Gen Psychiatry*, N0.64, pp. 830-842, ISSN 1538-3636

Heinz, A., Beck, A., Grusser, S.M., Grace, A.A. & Wrase J. (2009). Identifying the neural circuitry of alcohol craving and relapse vulnerability, *Addict Biol*, Vol.14, No.1, pp. 108-118, ISSN 1369-1600

Koob, G.F. (2000). Animal models of craving for ethanol. *Addiction*, Vol.95, Suppl.2, pp. s73-s81, ISSN 0965–2140

Koob, G.F. (2008). A role for brain stress systems in addiction, *Neuron*, Vol.59, N.1, pp. 11-34, ISSN 0896-6273

Koob, G.F. & Le Moal, M. (2008). Addiction and the Brain Antireward System, *Annu Rev Psychol*, Vol.59, pp. 29-53, ISSN 0066-4308

Liappas, J., Paparrigopoulos, E., Tzavellas, G. & Christodoulou G. (2002). Impact of alcohol detoxification on anxiety and depressive symptoms, *Drug Alcohol Depend*, No.68, pp. 215-220, ISSN 0376-8716

Mason, J.B., Light, M.J., Escher, T. & Drobes, J.D. (2008). Effects of positive and negative affective stimuli and beverage cues on measures of craving in non treatment-seeking alcoholics, *Psychopharmacology*, Vol.200, No.1, pp. 141-150, ISSN 1432-2072

Mendoza–Sassi, R. A. & Beria, J. U. (2003). Revalence of alcohol use disorders and associated factors: a population based study using AUDIT in southern Brazil, *Addiction*, Vol.98, No.6, pp. 799 – 804, ISSN 0965-2140

Miller, F., Miller, G., Miller, M., Knot, R. & Renn, W. (1994). *Breaking through denial – The SASSI a new addiction measure*, The SASSI Institute, Bloomington

Miller, W.R. & Tonigan, J.S. (1996). Assessing drinker's motivation for change: The stages of Change Readiness and Treatment Eagerness Scale (SOCRATES), *Psychology of Addiction Behaviors*, Vol.10, No.2, pp. 81-89, ISSN 0893-164X

Monti, P.M., Rohsenow, D.J. & Hutchison, K.E. (2000). Toward bridging the gap between biological, psychobiological and psychosocial models of alcohol craving, *Addiction*, Vol.95, Suppl 2, pp. s229-s236, ISSN 0965–2140

Oslin, D.W., Cary, M., Slaymaker, S., Colleran, C. & Blow, F.C. (2009). Daily ratings measures of alcohol craving during an inpatient stay define subtypes of alcohol addiction that predict subsequent risk for resumption of drinking, *Drug Alcohol Depen*, Vol.03, No.3, pp. 131-136, ISSN 0376-8716

Reinert, D.F. & Allen, J. P. (2002). The alcohol use disorders identification test (AUDIT): a review of recent research, *Alcohol Clin Exp Research*, Vol.26, No.2, pp. 272 – 279, ISSN 0145-6008

Sheehan, D.V., Lecrubier, Y., Sheehan, K.H., Amorim, P., Janavs, J., Weiller, E., Hergueta, T., Baker, R. & Dunbar, G.C. (1998). The Mini-International Neuropsychiatric Interview (M.I.N.I.): the development and validation of a structured diagnostic psychiatric interview for DSM-IV and ICD-10, *J Clin Psychiatry*, Vol.59, Suppl 20, pp. 22–33, ISSN 0160-6689

Spielberger, D.C., Gorsuch, R.L., Lushene, R., Vagg, P.R. & Jacobs, GA. (1983). *State-Trait Anxiety Inventory for Adult*, Manual, Test Booklet and Scoring Key. Consulting Psychologists Press, Mind Garden (sampler, received January 21, 2009)

Tiffany, S.T. (1990). A cognitive model of drug urges and drug-use behavior: Role of automatic and nonautomatic processes, *Psychological Review*, No.97, pp. 147-168, ISSN 0033-295X

Weegmann, M.(2002). The vulnerable self: Heinz Kohut and the addictions, in M. Weegmann & R. Cohen (eds.), *The psychodynamics of addiction*, Whurr Publishers, London and Philadelphia, pp. 31-50, ISBN 978 0 1 86156 335 4

Witkiewitz, K. & Bowen, S. (2010). Depression, Craving, and Substance Use Following a Randomized Trial of Mindfulness-Based Relapse Prevention, *J Consult Clin Psych*, Vol.78, No.3, pp. 362-374, ISSN 0022-006X

Witkiewitz, K., Bowen, S. & Donovan, D.M. (2011). Moderating Effect of a Intervention on the Relation Between Negative Mood and Heavy Drinking Following Treatment for Alcohol Dependence, *J Consult Clin Psych*, Vol.79, No.1, pp. 54-63, ISSN 0022-006X

Zung, W. (1965). A self-rating depression scale, *Arch Gen Psychiatry,No.* 12, pp. 63 – 70, ISSN 0003-990x

4

Workplace Functional Impairment Due to Mental Disorders

Charl Els, Diane Kunyk, Harold Hoffman and Adam Wargon
University of Alberta
Canada

1. Introduction

Psychiatrists are commonly expected to conduct disability assessments. These include an assessment of the worker's functioning, putative impairment, risk, and capacity to work. Employers and other third parties, either administrative or judicial, subsequently make disability determinations based on such assessments. This assessment also forms the foundation for return-to-work determinations, or for determining the employer's duty to accommodate to the point of undue hardship.

To the extent the general psychiatrist becomes involved in assessing these occupational matters, the psychiatrist is practicing forensic psychiatry. The role and responsibilities of the treating psychiatrist, within in the context of a traditional physician-patient relationship, differ vastly from one conducting an occupational or forensic evaluation. Yet, the boundaries between these distinct and often irreconcilable roles are not always clearly delineated, properly understood, or abided by. The forensic aspects of psychiatric practice are often viewed as intrusive and challenging by non-forensically trained psychiatrists, representing a role conflict many psychiatrists find themselves poorly equipped to navigate.

This chapter outlines the common psychiatric disorders encountered in clinical and occupational settings. It discusses the concepts of impairment and disability, as well as the benefits of working. The most commonly requested opinions in occupational psychiatric assessments are that of a psychiatric diagnosis, causation, impairment, fitness to work (FTW), and disability, along with recommendations for further investigations and treatment. The importance of objectively measuring impairment is outlined, along with reliably establishing a diagnosis (if any), along with the non-linear relationship between mental disorder, impairment and disability. For the purposes of this chapter, any reference to mental disorders are implied to include the broad range of disorders captured in the Diagnostic and Statistical Manual of Mental Disorders, the DSM IV-TR, which includes the substance-related disorders (i.e. Substance Abuse, Substance Dependence, or Addiction, and others, e.g. Addiction).

This chapter addresses the main pitfalls and risks associated with Independent Medical (i.e. Psychiatric and Addictions) Evaluations (IME), and provides a template for conducting these. The potential cost saving associated with implementing evidence-based interventions drives a sound business case for addressing mental disorders in the workplace. This chapter offers a pragmatic approach to treatment matching and disability management for workers with mental disorders (i.e. including substance-related disorders). It outlines the principles of vocational rehabilitation in the context of psychopathology, mental disorders, impairment and disability, ensuring safety, as well as optimal clinical and economic outcomes.

The enjoyment of the human right to optimal health, without discrimination, is vital to a person's well-being. This chapter aims to provide a pragmatic approach, albeit non-exhaustive, to determining mental impairment in the workplace.

2. The purpose of work

The Merriam-Webster dictionary defines *work* as "an activity in which one exerts strength of faculties to perform something: (a) sustained physical or mental effort to overcome obstacles and achieve an objective or result; (b) the labor, task, or duty that is one's accustomed means of livelihood; (c) a specific task, duty, or function, or assignment often being a part of phase of some larger activity".

Work plays a central role in daily life, and for most people, work is probably second only to love as a compelling human activity (O'Toole, 1982). Society values work and those who do, echoing the Latin phrase: "Labor corona vitae", loosely translated, "Work is life's crown". Working, gainfully or not, employed or not, may hold a range of psychological, monetary, and other potential benefits (Gold & Shuman, 2009):

1. Income and sense of security;
2. Source of identity, from which people derive a sense of recognition, belonging, and understanding;
3. Sense of purpose in life;
4. Source of self-worth and self-esteem;
5. Opportunity to develop skills and creativity;
6. Autonomy and independence;
7. Relationships outside the family;
8. Structuring time into predictable, regular periods;
9. Defines activities whereby work provides a temporal framework within which other activities, such as leisure, gain meaning.

The psychological benefits of work significantly overlap with several of the treatment goals in mental health settings. It suggests that employment has positive therapeutic benefits, but not all aspects of work are beneficial under all circumstances, or for every worker, e.g. where work causes inordinate levels of stress, or where a worker is exposed to discrimination or risks. Most workers do not become excessively distressed by the presence of challenges in their workplace, but rather by their inability to meet the particular challenge they are faced with (Aneshensel & Phelan, 1999).

Almost as a rule, the risk of exacerbating mental illness by returning workers to the workplace is minimal. Based on the evidence, return to work is generally stabilizing and therapeutic for the lives of these patients. In general, ongoing employment has a beneficial effect in persons with mental illness (Blustein, 2008). For the vast majority of workers, and under most circumstances, it is reasonable to suggest that active participation in work is therapeutic and beneficial.

3. Adopting a common language

Foundational to working with common psychopathology or mental disorders in the workplace is the use of common language. It is erroneous to use concepts like *impairment* and *disability* interchangeably. Failure to adequately and reliably delineate concepts of *risk*, *tolerance*, and *capacity* in the disability assessment, compromises a valid response to return-to-work determinations, the duty to accommodate, or further mental health disability management.

3.1 The definition of a "mental disorder"

Two major global classification systems provide a common language and standardized criteria for the diagnosis and classification of mental disorders. These are the 10th revision of the World Health Organization's (WHO) International Statistical Classification of Diseases and Related Health Problems (ICD-10) (WHO, 1992), and the 4th Edition (text-revised) of the American Psychiatric Association's (APA) Diagnostic and Statistical Manual of Mental Disorders (DSM IV-TR) (APA, 2000). There exists significant congruence between these two classification systems, with a reduction in differences between these two classification systems over time.

For the purposes of this chapter, the authors will utilize the DSM as the predominant classification system and frame of reference in the authors' jurisdiction. Since the publication of the first edition of the DSM in 1952, the manual has undergone vast changes, and the manual is currently in its 4th edition, of which the text has been revised. The DSM-5 is expected within the next 2 years, updating the current DSM IV-TR, describing almost 300 mental disorders, which includes the categories of substance-related disorders (i.e. substance use disorders, e.g. abuse and dependence, and the substance-induced disorders).

The terms *illness, disease,* and *disorder,* as it pertains to the mental (psychiatric) status of the worker, are often used interchangeably. For the purposes of this chapter, the term *disorder* is preferred, defined as a *"deviation from the normal or expected status, associated with distress or a deterioration in functionality".* The term *mental* refers to *"(a) inner experiences, relating to mood, thought content, or sensory experiences; (b) behavioral patterns, and (c) cognitive functions such as learning, social understanding, and reality assessment",* and a *mental disorder* is conceptualized in the DSM IV-TR (APA, 2000) as a *"clinically significant behavioral or psychological pattern that occurs in an individual and that is associated with present distress (e.g. a painful symptom) or disability (i.e. impairment in one or more important areas of functioning) or with a significantly increased risk of suffering death, pain, disability, or an important loss of freedom".* The concept of mental disorder does not include a situation that is merely an expectable and culturally sanctioned response to events, e.g. the emotional response of bereavement following a significant loss, e.g. the death of a loved one.

Symptoms and signs of mental disorders may include any combination of affective, behavioral, cognitive, and perceptual components. To allow for consistency of diagnosis, standardized criteria are outlined in the DSM, based on the best available research and clinical literature. Illegal or deviant behavior and conflict (i.e. primarily between the individual and society) are not considered mental disorders unless this actually represents a symptom of dysfunction in the individual. Mental disorders are a rarely cause of unlawful behavior or violence.

Mental disorders are diagnoses representing syndromes, based on clusters of symptoms and signs, as opposed to many other medical conditions with consistent and proven underlying pathophysiology. It utilizes a categorical approach where there exists no assumption that each category of mental disorder is completely discrete from other mental disorders, or that there exist absolute boundaries dividing disorders from one another. The diagnostic criteria, albeit based on consensus of current formulations of evolving knowledge in the field, do not encompass all the conditions for which persons may be treated (APA, 2000).

3.2 The 5-Axis formulation

The DSM system has gained wide international acceptance and the 5-Axis description is deemed a gold standard for offering a standardized psychiatric formulation, across international borders and cultural boundaries. To standardize the approach for occupational assessments, the 5 Axes formulation is also considered an essential component of formulating the results of the assessment:

Axis I: Clinical Disorder(s)
               Other condition(s) that may be a focus of clinical attention
Axis II: Personality Disorder(s)
               Mental Retardation
Axis III: General Medical Condition(s)
Axis IV: Psychosocial and Environmental Problem(s)
Axis V: Global Assessment of Functioning (GAF)

The use of *specifiers* assists in further describing the specific diagnosis on Axis I. If criteria are met for a specific mental disorder, severity may be specified as mild or moderate or severe, and if criteria are no longer met, a specifier for remission may be offered, e.g. in partial remission, in full remission, or suggesting a "prior history" of the disorder existed.

On Axis V, the GAF rating offers a dimensional assessment of overall functioning, but which is not only indicative of occupational functioning. The scoring for Axis V is divided into 10 ranges of functioning, and reflects the clinician's judgment of the respondent's overall level of functioning. It is useful in monitoring impact of treatment, and also in predicting treatment outcome (APA, 2000). Although the adjudication of insurance claims takes GAF scoring into consideration, it should not be the sole determinant of fitness-to-work. The GAF score, albeit useful, is not specific to fitness-to-work. Utilizing GAF scores alone to determine fitness-to-work should be avoided.

3.3 Expressing a degree of uncertainty

In determining if a worker fulfills the diagnostic criteria for a specific mental disorder, a certain degree of uncertainty may prevail. These include situations where inadequate information is available for making an accurate diagnostic judgment. In other situations limited information may be available, perhaps only sufficient to determine and validate the presence of a *class* of disorders (e.g. mood disorder, psychotic disorder, anxiety disorder), but where further specification of the particular disorder within the class is not possible. In other cases information may be altogether inadequate to offer any diagnosis whatsoever. Under these circumstances where a formal diagnosis cannot be offered with a reasonable level of certainty, the situation may call for a proper description of the level of uncertainty. The use of terms to describe these levels of uncertainty include the following: offering a *provisional* diagnosis, *deferring* a diagnosis, offering the diagnosis of an *unspecified* mental disorder, or of a mental disorder "*not otherwise specified*" (NOS). As a result of the limitations of this categorical (as opposed to a dimensional) approach, in some cases the diagnosis of a mental disorder can only be offered in a probabilistic fashion.

3.4 Limitations in the use of the classification system in occupational context

The categorical approach to diagnosis of mental illness poses challenges in quantifying mental and behavioral impairment in a dimensional fashion. Mental disorders, in the absence of the currently proven underlying pathophysiology and absent operational definition, have been defined by a variety of concepts, e.g. distress, dysfunction, dyscontrol, disadvantage, disability, inflexibility, irrationality, syndromal pattern, etiology, and statistical deviation (APA, 2000). These levels of abstraction do not constitute a consistent or equivalent description of any one specific mental disorder in any single class.

Relying on the diagnosis alone does not provide sufficient evidence of the existence of impairment or disability. The levels of abstraction appear on a continuum of severity, and no single diagnosis of a mental disorder automatically implies a universal or specific level of impairment, or a specific degree of disability.

Volatility, interpersonal conflict, and unreliability are also relevant to fitness for work. These may be unrelated to mental disorders, and may hence not qualify as compensable conditions under disability determination paradigms used by a third party. Further, the inclusion of diagnostic categories (e.g. antisocial personality disorder, pedophilia) does not imply that the specific condition meets the *legal* criteria for what constitutes a mental disorder.

The determination of the level of functional impairment faces significant impediments: the disturbance in functional activities is driven by the diagnosis and not test results per se. For example, a diagnosis alone does not determine fitness for work – just as the diagnosis of diabetes is not necessarily limiting to work under certain circumstances. But, uncontrolled diabetes poses a risk for work, especially in safety-sensitive settings. In the absence of external validation, there exists a potential for large inter-individual variability in interpretation of levels of impairment or disability associated with a mental disorder. There are few objective measures to ensure reliability and validity of impairment ratings. The dearth of validated tests to confirm the percentage of psychiatric impairment and the apportionment due to mental disorders, poses a salient challenge.

The use of the DSM in forensic settings should be conducted with caution, as the categorization of disorders in clinical and research context may not take into account the necessary issues of responsibility, competence, tolerance, risk, or disability. Blindly relying only on the DSM diagnostic criteria poses a significant risk that the clinical information may be misused or erroneously interpreted by a third party that does not take into account any level of clinical judgment. The classification system is ultimately intended to serve only as a guideline to be informed by clinical judgment and are not meant to be used in a "cookbook fashion" (APA, 2000). The establishment of a DSM IV-TR diagnosis represents only the first step in a more comprehensive evaluation. This is the basis for further assessment or treatment planning may rest, and also upon which disability management or accommodation may be based.

3.4 Impairment *versus* disability

The AMA Guides to the Evaluation of Permanent Impairment, Sixth Edition (AMA, 2011) defines *impairment* and *disability*. Impairment refers to "*a significant deviation, loss, or loss of use of any body structure or body function in an individual with a health condition, disorder, or disease.*" Impairment rating is a physician-provided process that attempts to link impairment with functional loss. It is also a "*consensus-derived percentage estimate of loss of activity reflecting severity for a given health condition, and the degree of associated limitations in terms of activities of daily living*". Impairment ratings are conducted by the physician, whereas disability assessments are conducted by the third party.

Disability refers to "*activity limitations and/or participation restrictions in an individual with a health condition, disorder, or disease.*" The disability determination takes into account the lack or restriction in the ability to perform an activity in the manner or within the range of what is deemed normal or expected. Impairment and disability fall on a spectrum of low to high severity. The determination of disability is thus a relational outcome, contingent upon the environment in which the particular demands are met, by a specific individual, based on the activities performed, within a specific occupational environment. The level of disability is dependent on the relational aspects or interplay between impairment and several factors within the occupational environment.

Regardless of the diagnosis, the relationship between impairment, disability, and fitness to work depends on the respondent's functional abilities and functional limitations, the occupational environment, and the specific demands of any particular job (Bonnie 1997; Gold and Shuman 2009). Not all individuals with psychopathology or mental disorders necessarily display significant impairment or disability, despite the presence of diagnosable DSM conditions. Similarly, not all persons displaying mental disorders are necessarily deemed disabled based on the presence of a psychiatric disorder. No linear relationship exists to predict the level of impairment or disability associated with any particular mental disorder. Return to work depends on availability of modified work, job skills, and medical limitations.

3.5 "*Presenteeism*" and absenteeism

Absenteeism refers to repeated absence from work, duties, or obligations. *Presenteeism* refers to a situation where the employee is present at work, but not functioning at full capacity, or at a lower level of productivity, as a result of a mental disorder or psychopathology. Both presenteeism and absenteeism may be indicative of employer performance issues, workplace issues, employer issues, relational issues between employer and employee, or of a medical or psychiatric impairment and subsequent inability to perform in the expected fashion, or the incurring of risks. More than 80% of lost productivity and associated cost related to mental disorders is accounted for by *presenteeism* as opposed to absenteeism.

3.6 The concepts of risk, capacity, and tolerance

Commonly requested occupational psychiatric opinions pertain to that of risk assessment, tolerance, and capacity. *Risk* refers to the potential for a specific situation to translate into negative outcomes, including accidents, lack of attention, violence, injury (patient, coworkers, public, or equipment), or aggressive behavior. The risk may result from specific actions or inactions by the employer, and is confounded by a range of factors of which the class of substance used disorders is a salient predictor of violence, especially when co-occurring with mental illness.

Aggressive behavior constituting increased risk ranges from minor incidents to more significant behavioral actions and disturbances, including homicide, suicide, assault, terrorism (e.g. some industrial settings may be at risk of such attacks) or the damaging of property. Certain mental disorders are more likely to be associated with increased risk, i.e. the psychotic disorders, individuals with a previous risk of harm to self or others, those with a previous history of aggressive behavior, those with comorbid mental disorders and substance use disorders, those with paranoia or homicidal or suicidal ideation, persons with antisocial personality disorders, or any combination of such factors. Risk assessments trump most other considerations in the assessment.

Capacity refers to the employee's ability to perform or to produce according to occupational expectations. Mental disorders and substance use disorders can impact on the employee's memory, the ability to concentrate, focusing attention, and on judgment, fatigue, insomnia, tendency to fall asleep, and decreased reaction (e.g. truck driver, pilot, or police) Medical conditions, mental disorders, substance use disorders, or any combination of these, including the adverse effects of medications, may adversely impact on the employee's performance and may pose safety risks.

Tolerance addresses the employee's ability and/or willingness to tolerate (accept or similar word) the workplace and associated circumstances and stressors. The most prominent factor in this context refers to motivation (representing an inner state) to return to work, or to perform in the workplace. Motivation is impacted by the respondent's appraisal of the relative importance to perform particular duties according to standards and expectations, paired with the relative confidence that he/she would be able to do so. It represents a predominantly volitional state of choice in terms of what the employee chooses to tolerate and what the worker chooses not to tolerate. Difficulties in the workplace, including unreasonable workload demands, job dissatisfaction, suboptimal goodness-of-fit, job changes, relational and interpersonal problems with co-workers or supervisors, negative evaluations or warning letters, or threat of layoff or termination, may foreseeably impact or contribute to the subjective distress. These, however, have to be separated from bona fide mental disorders in causing subjective distress or functional impairment.

Workplace issues may contribute to symptoms, but are not considered causally related to bona fide psychiatric illness or disability as a result of a mental disorder e.g. when a worker is disciplined for performance issues, the expected response is to react with a sense of subjective distress, like feeling depressed, anxious, frustrated, or angry. This is, however, to be distinguished from bona fide symptoms related to a psychiatric disorder in adjudicating disability matters. When an employer or supervisor disciplines a worker for performance issues, then the worker often claims stress or depression attributed to this event. Workplace stress and burnout are commonly attributed to the workplace. Post-Traumatic Stress Disorder (PTSD) from life-threatening events at work may plausibly cause impairment, preclude fitness for duty, and legitimately lead to disability.

3.7 Restrictions and limitations

An integral part of the occupational assessment concerns itself with the determination if the worker's psychiatric clinical condition is severe enough to limit or restrict their ability to perform occupational functions. In general, *restrictions* refer to activities / duties the worker "should not do", while *limitations* describe as what a worker "cannot do" due to severity of psychiatric impairment. Fitness to work-related terms are described as follows: a. Capabilities (i.e. the maximum that this person can do); b. Limitations (i.e. this person cannot do more than this); and c. Restrictions (i.e. this person can do this, but should not do this).

4. Causality of the workplace in the development of impairment

There exist no single or definitive model for understanding the etiology and pathology of mental disorders. Psychopathology and mental disorders stem from a variety of origins, and vary widely across disorders and classes. A variety of hypotheses have been postulated to explain the origins of mental disorders, and these theories continue to evolve. Some of the most common perspectives for the understanding of psychopathology and etiology of mental disorders include: (1) neurobiological, (2) sociobiological, (3) psychodynamic, (4) behavioristic, (5) cognitive, (6) interpersonal and systems, (7) humanistic, and (8) anthropological (Thomas & Hersen, 2004). The stress-diathesis and bio-psycho-social models offer two of the more generic approaches to understanding respectively the significant roles of stress and the role of biological, psychological, and social factors play in human functioning as well as in the development of illness or disorders (Engel, 1977). None of these categories suggest participation in work per se to be psychopathogenic, i.e. causing psychiatric disorders or psychopathology.

Working, unlike the commonly understood etiological factors, is not viewed as a risk factor and therefore also not a cause of the development of a mental disorder or substance-related disorder. Despite common claims made by workers suffering from mental disorders, there is a lack of definitive empirical evidence to suggest that employment is a causal factor in the development of mental disorders. In determining the etiology, it is commonly understood that non-occupational factors are overwhelmingly deemed as causal and relevant agents in the development of mental disorders. In other words, work does not cause mental illness or addiction, but work rather protects against the development of mental disorders. When a worker is disciplined, or where workplace issues may exist, a worker may claim "stress" or attempt to attribute depression (or a mental disorder) as a result of these events in the workplace. Workplace stress and burnout are commonly attributed to the workplace, despite the dearth of empirical evidence to support a direct and causal relationship. Where the treating physician becomes involved in offering opinions or conclusions related to disability, the role of the advocating physician might obfuscate the adjudication of a claim.

There are legitimate occupational causes for mental disorders, e.g. where an individual has been exposed to a significant or life-threatening stressor (e.g. where he/she feared for life), PTSD may develop.

5. Psychopathology and psychiatric disorders in the workplace

5.1 Prevalence of mental disorders and disability in the workplace

Over a third of people in most countries report meeting criteria for the major categories of either mental illness or addiction, or both at some point in their lives. Psychiatric impairment and disability may be associated with a broad range of psychiatric disorders, and may be debilitating under some circumstances. Disability is a common, though uniquely personal experience, with an estimated 15% of the world's population thought to have a disability.

Most of the empirical work to date focused on persons with Mood Disorders (Major Depressive Disorder, Bipolar Disorder), Anxiety disorders (specifically Generalized Anxiety Disorder (GAD), and Post-Traumatic Stress Disorder (PTSD), the psychotic disorders (specifically Schizophrenia), Personality Disorders, Substance Use Disorders (Substance Abuse and Substance Dependence), the functional somatic syndromes (e.g. Somatoform Disorders). These disorders represent the mental disorders most commonly found in occupational settings and comorbidity (i.e. co-occurrence of psychiatric illnesses) is common. The prevalence of commonly encountered workplace psychiatric disorders by class and specific diagnosis is reflected in Table 1 (Kessler, Berglund, et al., 2005; Kessler, Chiu, et al., 2005).

The majority of individuals with psychopathology and mental disorders continue to be employed. The presence of a mental disorder does not automatically preclude an individual from working safely and successfully. In general, however, severe and persistent mental illness (SPMI) tends to be more likely disabling, e.g. Bipolar Disorder and Schizophrenia. The worker who suffers from at least one SPMI is often are unable to compete on equal footing for employment, and hence SPMI is rarely encountered in most occupational settings. The less severe mental disorders do not typically preclude individuals from competing for employment, and are hence seen more commonly in occupational settings.

Class of Disorder	Specific Diagnosis	Lifetime Prevalence (%)	12-month prevalence (%)
Anxiety Disorders		28.8	18.1
	Panic Disorder	4.7	2.7
	Specific Phobia	12.5	8.7
	Social Phobia	12.1	6.8
	Generalized Anxiety Disorder	5.7	3.1
	Post-traumatic Stress Disorder	6.8	3.5
	Obsessive Compulsive Disorder	1.6	1.0
Mood Disorders		20.8	9.5
	Major Depressive Disorder	16.6	6.7
	Dysthymia	2.5	1.5
	Bipolar I and II	3.9	2.6
Impulse Control Disorders			
	Attention deficit / hyperactivity Disorder	8.1	4.1
Substance Use Disorders		14.6	3.8
	Alcohol Use	13.2	3.1
	Alcohol Dependence	5.4	1.3
	Drug Use	7.9	1.4
	Drug Dependence	3.0	0.4

Table 1.

5.2 Major Depressive Disorder (MDD)

Major Depressive Disorder (MDD) is often a common and chronic condition, with a lifetime risk of 10-25% for women and 5-12% for men, in community-based settings. The essential feature of MDD is a clinical course that is characterized by one or more Major Depressive Episodes (APA, 2000). Major Depressive Episodes may occur in the context of MDD or Bipolar I or II Disorder. The MDE in a MDD has to be distinguished from legitimate stress related to workplace issues, a depressed mood related to substance use, (i.e. Substance-Induced Mood Disorder, e.g. with the use of alcohol or cocaine and other drugs), and a Mood Disorder due to a General Medical Condition, e.g. where hypothyroidism is responsible for symptoms of a mood disorder.

The use of the term "depression" to describe the mental disorder diagnosis is inappropriate as it represents only one symptom of a syndrome, by itself does not reliably describe a specific mental disorder. The diagnostic criteria for MDE and MDD, as well as other disorders associated with a depressed mood are captured in the DSM IV-TR (APA, 2000). The term "clinical depression" is no longer recommended for use, and for the diagnosis of MDD a range of specifiers allow for finer description of the disorder, e.g. severity (i.e. mild, moderate, or severe). There also exist remission specifiers, i.e. partial or full remission, as well as specifiers to indicate the presence of catatonic features, psychotic features, melancholic features, atypical features, or with post-partum onset. Course specifiers, i.e. with or without interepisode recovery, or with seasonal pattern allows for longitudinal descriptions, along with the descriptors of single episode, recurrent, and chronic. Dysthymic Disorder refers to a disorder associated with a chronically depressed mood or irritability that occurs for most days for at least two years, upon which a MDD could be superimposed. There are no diagnostic laboratory tests for any of the depressive disorders, but non-specific findings have been described, e.g. elevated glucocorticoid levels as well as EEG sleep alterations. Because up to a quarter of persons with certain medical conditions will develop depression (APA, 2000), medical conditions and substance-related disoders have to be ruled out in any person diagnosed with a MDE.

Depressive disorders are considered a leading cause of disability globally (Murray & Lopez, 1996), projected to become the world's leading cause of disability. Most persons with mild depression can continue to function in the workplace, despite the presence of some degree of impairment or the presence of related symptoms. In those suffering from one or more depressive disorder absenteeism and presenteeism are linked to decreased productivity and an increased potential for risk in some, as a direct result of the symptoms (both physical and mental) of depression. These include depressed mood, irritability, low energy, cognitive symptoms (attention, memory, distractibility, executive function) and loss of motivation, or thoughts of death, dying, and suicide. Like in the case with other mental disorders, the mere presence of the diagnosis of MDD is not an indication of the level of impairment. The DSM IV-TR criteria require to be supplemented with a dimensional functional assessment to determine the level of impairment, based on which disability determinations should be based.

A number of substance-related disorders may mimic the features of MDD and other disorders in this class, and require to be ruled out in the diagnosis of the condition. These include mood disorders that develop as the direct result of the use of alcohol, amphetamines, cocaine, hallucinogens, inhalants, opioids, sedatives / hypnotics, or any combination thereof, i.e. poly-substance use. The condition of a depressive episode may be mimicked in either intoxication or withdrawal phases of substance use, and may be compounded by the presence of a bona fide medical condition.

Clinical practice guidelines for the treatment of MDD typically include multimodal pharmacotherapy and psychotherapy combinations. In the management of MDD, attention should be given to the detection and treatment not only of the primary condition, but also of comorbidity of any substance-related disorder, specifically Alcohol Abuse or Dependence, as well as the potential for imminent risk of harm to self or to others. With the appropriate treatment, 80% of depressed individuals can return to normal activities, including work. Improvements following treatment initiation are usually notable within 10 days to 2 weeks, and with relatively rapid improvement in work function. Adverse effects of antidepressants are usually evident within the first two weeks, and in general these are mild and transient. In the face of untreated depression, chronicity may develop, with subsequent increased levels of disability as a result of chronic impairments.

Because MDD and other depressive disorders may be associated with an increased risk of harm to self, the necessary level of vigilance is required to detect any safety risk in occupational context.

5.3 Bipolar Disorder

Bipolar I Disorder is ranked as a leading cause of disability, but is less prevalent than MDD. As a result of the heterogeneous nature of this disorder, workers can present with a variety of symptoms, e.g. depressed, hypomania (Bipolar II Disorder), mania (Bipolar I Disorder), or psychotic features (i.e. hallucinations, delusions, disorganized behavior). The condition is typically characterized by the presence of chronic symptoms, either mania, or depression, or both in alternating or mixed cycles. The diagnosis of Bipolar Disorder also warrants the rigorous exclusion of any substance-related disorder as the clinical presentation of this condition may be mimicked by a number of substance use disorders, e.g. alcohol, stimulants (e.g. cocaine, crystal methamphetamine), and over-the-counter medications. The impairment related to Bipolar I Disorder will depend on the phase of the illness the worker is in as well as the relative intensity of the symptoms, e.g. cognitive symptoms during the depressive phase, as opposed to disinhibition during the manic phase of the disorder.

Bipolar Disorder is considered chronic, yet treatable, but treatment is generally more complex than for MDD, and closer attention is given to treatment adherence. The utilization of multimodal interventions, i.e. including mood stabilizers and psychotherapy, along with longitudinal follow-up by an attending physician, is deemed the mainstay of treatment. Although considered treatable, the course of the disorder is typically recurrent and more than half of persons diagnosed with the disorder continue to experience interpersonal or occupational difficulties between acute episodes. As a general statement, the prognosis for Bipolar I Disorder is less optimistic than for MDD, and approximately 10-15% of persons diagnosed with Bipolar I Disorder complete suicide.

A number of substance use disorders may mimic the features of Bipolar Disorder, and requires to be ruled out in the diagnosis of the condition. These include: alcohol, amphetamines, cocaine, hallucinogens, inhalants, opioids, and poly-substance use.

5.4 Anxiety Disorders

On a daily basis, most persons in the general population will experience varying degrees of anxiety. This is necessary for survival and tends to increase performance, and is not considered pathological. However, when the threshold for a disorder is reached (i.e. causing significant distress or leading to significant functional impairment), and the DSM criteria are met, an Anxiety Disorder is diagnosed. Anxiety Disorders are the most common psychiatric disorders, and may be associated with significant impairment. This class of disorders includes Generalized Anxiety Disorder (GAD), Post-Traumatic Stress Disorder (PTSD), Acute Stress Disorder, Social Anxiety Disorder (Social Phobia), Panic Disorder with / without Agoraphobia, Agoraphobia without a history of Panic Disorder, Specific Phobias, Obsessive-Compulsive Disorder (OCD), Anxiety Disorder due to a General Medical Condition, and Substance-Induced Anxiety Disorder. While low levels of anxiety is ubiquitous and may increase productivity, it may equally be potentially impairing when it exceeds threshold levels.

There is no direct correlation between any single Anxiety Disorder, the level of impairment, fitness to work and subsequent disability. The complex relationship requires the assessment of the individual, with measurement of the level of functioning and the putative impairment as a result of the condition. Panic attacks and PTSD tend to be most disabling, and special attention should be given to ruling out medical conditions or substance use patterns that may mimic anxiety, or substances, which may be used to self-medicate anxiety symptoms.

Anxiety Disorders are highly treatable, with multimodal interventions, including pharmacotherapy and psychotherapy. The response to medication in the context of OCD may take longer than for other anxiety disorders, and higher dosages may be required compared to other disorders in the same class. Caution should be taken with regards to the use of sedating or habit-forming classes of medication for the treatment of the worker with an Anxiety Disorder, as it may increase the risk of cognitive impairment, the risk of accidents (specifically in safety-sensitive positions), or it may provoke complications with regards to other addictive disorders (e.g. in a person with pre-existing history of problem related to among others alcohol, barbiturates, opioid, or benzodiazepines).

5.5 Substance-related disorders

The impact of substances on the workplace is diverse and potentially severe, posing salient safety concerns for those working in safety-sensitive occupations. The essential feature of Substance Dependence (addiction) is a cluster of cognitive, behavioral, and physiological symptoms indicating that the individual continues use of the substance despite significant substance-related problems (APA, 2000). Eleven classes of substances are listed in the DSM, including alcohol, amphetamines, caffeine, cannabis, cocaine, hallucinogens, inhalants, nicotine, opioids, phencyclidine, sedatives-hypnotics or anxiolytics, and there is allowance for poly-substance use as well. The use of caffeine and nicotine are generally not deemed impairing in the short-term, although the chronic use of tobacco is an obvious and common cause of death, disease, and medical disability.

Although the use of substances is ubiquitous in the general population, only a fraction of those who use drugs are deemed as suffering from a mental disorder, i.e. Substance Abuse or Dependence. Substance abuse disorders can be associated with lifestyle changes, such as socializing at bars or having business meetings in facilities where alcohol is served. The use of substances may be used recreationally and in a non-addictive pattern, or the user may become addicted to it. Substance use, whether used recreationally or in the context of having become addicted, poses significant concerns to persons working in safety-sensitive occupations. Ongoing substance use in a worker who has ever been diagnosed with Substance Abuse or Dependence (excluding nicotine) is generally inconsistent with functioning in a safety-sensitive position. Total abstinence of all classes of drugs of abuse (excluding nicotine) is usually required under such circumstances, to avoid the potential impact ongoing use may have.

The impact of substances on performance and safety in the workplace goes beyond the immediate intoxicating effects of the substance, may also be related to withdrawal symptoms, and also to carry-over effects of certain drugs that are used outside working hours. An additional and significant factor for the worker consuming illicit substances is that the person must purchase the substance by illegal methods, and this requires the worker to have contacts with individuals engaging in criminal activity. This exposes the worker to a range of potential complications, associated with the subculture in which trafficking occurs.

Apart from the acute effects of drugs during intoxication and withdrawal, chronic drug use, especially alcohol, may also be associated with cerebral atrophy and cognitive deficits. Many psychiatric disorders are associated with an increased risk for Substance Abuse, and comorbidity has to be ruled out. This suggests that an individual undergoing a psychiatric assessment should be assessed for substance use issues, and vice versa. The request for an "addiction assessment" in the expressed absence of any psychiatric assessment represents a potential ethical quandary, which may impact on safety as well as the adjudication of any disability claim.

5.6 Personality disorders

The DSM IV-TR defines Personality Disorder (PD), as applied to the 10 specific Personality Disorders: *"An enduring pattern of inner experience and behavior that deviates markedly from the expectations of the individual's culture, is pervasive and inflexible, has an onset in adolescence or early adulthood, is stable over time, and leads to distress or impairment"* (APA, 2000). The Personality Disorders are divided into three Clusters: A, B, and C. Individuals in Cluster A (Paranoid PD, Schizoid PD, and Schizotypal PD) appear odd or eccentric, while individuals in Cluster B (Antisocial PD, Borderline PD, Histrionic PD, and Narcissistic PD) appear dramatic, emotional, or erratic. Persons in Cluster C (Avoidant PD, Dependent PD, Obsessive-Compulsive PD) often appear anxious and fearful (APA, 2000).

In this category the DSM includes the following disorders, with descriptions offered from the same source:

- Paranoid Personality Disorder: (referring to a pattern of distrust and suspiciousness such that others' motives are interpreted as malevolent);
- Schizoid Personality Disorder: (a pattern of detachment from social relationships and a restricted range of emotional expression);
- Schizotypal Personality Disorder: (a pattern of acute discomfort in close relationships, cognitive or perceptual distortions, and eccentricities of behavior);
- Antisocial Personality Disorder: (a pattern of disregard for, and violation of, the rights of others);
- Borderline Personality Disorder: (a pattern of instability in interpersonal relationships, self-image, and affect, and marked impulsivity);
- Histrionic Personality Disorder: (a pattern of excessive emotionality and attention-seeking);
- Narcissistic Personality Disorder: (a pattern of grandiosity, need for admiration, and lack of empathy);
- Avoidant Personality Disorder: (a pattern of social inhibition, feelings of inadequacy, and hypersensitivity to negative evaluation);
- Dependent Personality Disorder: (a pattern of submissive and clinging behavior related to an excessive need to be taken care of);
- Obsessive-compulsive Personality Disorder: (a pattern of preoccupation with orderliness, perfection, and control)
- Personality Disorder Not Otherwise Specified: (this section is reserved for situations where the person's personality meets the general criteria for a Personality Disorder and the traits of several Personality Disorders are present, but the criteria for any one specific Personality Disorder are not met).

Although persons with Personality Disorders may legitimately suffer from symptoms and signs, which may constitute impairment, these disorders (in the absence of Axis I disorders) would generally not be deemed compensable in disability adjudication processes. Individuals with personality disorders may experience a lack of goodness-of-fit in the context of their occupational situation, and issues are often dealt with in a performance fashion as opposed to an accommodation paradigm.

6. The cost of mental health disability

Common psychiatric disorders, including Addiction, frequently lead to an inability to work and contribute to both visible and invisible costs of disability (Armstrong, 2008). The invisible costs associated with not treating mental disorders in the workplace include loss of productivity, absenteeism, presenteeism, and the inability to retain a worker, i.e. leading to increased employee turn-over. Globally, mental disorders rank among the most common workplace disabilities. The key drivers of increasing disability costs are psychiatric disabilities or mental disorders. Mental disorders are the leading cause of long-term disability (72%) and short-term disability (82%), representing about 12% of overall Canadian business payroll costs (Watson Wyatt, 2007). Indirect costs of mental illnesses account for about 75% of total employer costs (McCulloch et al., 2001). The 2001 Health Canada report "The Economic Burden of Mental Health Problems in Canada" estimates the cost of lost productivity due to depression and stress at more than $8.1 billion dollars a year (Stephens & Joubert, 2001).

7. The occupational mental health assessment

7.1 Dual agents and advocacy bias

The World Medical Association reminds treating physicians that they have an ethical duty and a professional responsibility to act in the best interest of their patients without regard to age, gender, sexual orientation, physical ability or disability, race, religion, culture, beliefs, political affiliation, financial means or nationality (WMA, 2006).

Often a conflict emerges between the patient's legitimate health interests and the third party's specific requirements. When conducting independent assessments, the expectations from the patient and the treating physician are not always or necessarily aligned with those of the employer, insurer, regulatory, or legal system (collectively termed "third party"). Situations arise where there exists a conflict between the interest of the patient (and whereby the treating physician is obligated to act as a patient advocate, or where the duty dictates that the physician should act in the best interest of the patient) and the third party, whose decisions are typically shaped by economic, administrative, occupational, or legal parameters. It is considered a failure to meet professional standards as well as an ethical violation for a treating physician to offer conclusions about causation and other forensic issues (Greenberg & Shuman, 1997; Hales & Yudofsky, 2002; Barth & Brigham, 2005, Talmage, et al, 2011).

Under all circumstances, the independent assessment boundaries should clearly communicate (in advance) that the assessing physician has no duty to advocate for the patient (respondent). The duty also exists to communicate that the assessing psychiatrist is not employed by, or otherwise affiliated with, the retaining third party. If an assessing physician has previously provided treatment to the worker who has to be assessed, or has other affiliation with the retaining third party, the assessment is no longer deemed independent and the results may not be valid. To avoid these pitfalls, clear boundaries should be communicated in advance of the commencement of the assessment.

Attempting to fulfill both services and roles for the same worker (who has to be assessed) represents a conflict of interest for the psychiatrist and represents an ethical conundrum. These concerns pertaining to acting as dual agents should be addressed with the party in violation of the guideline. Psychiatrists acting as treatment providers should avoid offering opinions and conclusions pertaining to fitness-to-work, causation, or other forensic matters. It is however, permissible for the treating health professional to offer content witness input, but should avoid acting in both capacities.

7.2 The setting in which the Independent Medical Examination (IME) is conducted

The typical IME is conducted on an elective outpatient basis. The office setting deemed suitable for general psychiatric practice is usually suitable for conducting an IME. The reliance on usual protective measures to ensure safety is recommended. The assessment usually takes longer than a regular clinical assessment, and is not routinely audio/video-recorded unless the request for such is made in advance. The presence of a collateral source is not encouraged, but is not disallowed if requested.

7.3 Issues related to consent for obtaining or release of information

In an IME, the examining psychiatrist is responsible to explain the parameters, scope, risks, and who receives the report. This function, like obtaining consent, should not be delegated to office staff. The health professional conducting the independent assessment has an ethical and legal obligation to ensure that respondents are informed of their legal rights with respect to the assessment service (in this case referring to the occupational assessment, which is a forensic assessment). The respondent is advised that a traditional physician-patient relationship is not established, and that no duty to advocate or engage in a longitudinal therapeutic relationship is implied. This limited physician-patient relationship is subject to compliance to the same ethical principles as a traditional therapeutic relationship, in that objectivity needs to be achieved, the highest degree of confidentiality needs to be maintained, potential conflicts of interest should be declared, and boundaries should be honored (i.e. adherence to the same rules strictly proscribing boundary violations).

The respondent has to be informed of the purposes and parameters of the evaluation, of the nature of procedures to be employed, of the intended uses of any product of the assessing physician's services, and of the party who has retained the assessing professional. To protect confidentiality, the employer is typically entitled only to the fitness-to-work information (as opposed to the entire clinical assessment), while the disability manager may have access to the entire data set. Although the employer is not entitled to receive information pertaining to the exact diagnosis, it is not unusual for the employer to demand the full independent report. This conflict is resolved by attempting to utilize the services of a separate health professional (e.g. Occupational Health Nurse) as the designated employer representative. This person then acts as a caretaker of the information (in order for the non-relevant clinical and personal information to not go to Human Resources, the Employer, or beyond), but to remain in the hands of a health professional.

The worker should understand the lack of confidentiality in regards to anything discussed during the assessment, as it would potentially form part of the assessment report, which is communicated to the retaining third party, i.e. the employer or its designate. The results of any blood testing or urine drug screening should be incorporated into the report as deemed necessary to provide a reliable and valid independent opinion, and the worker should be fully informed and unless valid consent is obtained, such assessment cannot proceed. Only under the circumstances under which the worker fully understands the nature of the assessment, as well as his/her legal rights, could consent be viewed as valid. In the absence of valid consent, the assessment cannot proceed. Valid consent statements should be included in the report to the third party, and an example of such statement is as follows:

"Mr. John Doe was advised to the purpose and parameters of this assessment, as well as to the lack of confidentiality in regards to anything discussed, as it would potentially form part of the assessment. Mr. Doe was also informed that the information would be sent to the requester of this report, and that the results of any blood testing or urine drug screen would be incorporated into the report. Mr. Doe

was notified and understood that this would be an independent assessment, initially requested by a third party, and that a retainer was initiated by the third party. However, there existed no other affiliation with such, or with her employer, and the writer confirmed that he had not previously provided health services to him. Mr. Doe was also notified that this assessment would constitute a single liaison, which did not, and would not in future, constitute the establishment of a physician-patient relationship. As the writer, I notified Mr. Doe that I could not release a copy of this report to him, but that he would be able to approach the retaining third party regarding the protocols for obtaining a copy of this report. The writer also has no objection if a copy of this report is to be shared with any of the attending health professionals, with the appropriate consent as needed. Mr. Doe was given the ongoing opportunity to ask questions regarding the assessment, and was satisfied with the parameters of this protocol, and fully complied with the entire assessment. Upon request, he furnished the writer of this report with a government-issued proof of identification. There were no issues with language competence or understanding".

In situations where the respondent is unable to furnish the assessing party with a reasonable form of picture identification, the assessment report should include a detailed description of the respondent to ensure that the person assessed was indeed the individual under discussion and referred for assessment. If there are issues with language competence, the duty of the assessor is to wait until adequate interpretation services to be utilized. The responsibility for such falls on the shoulders of the retaining third party.

7.4 Duty to report

In certain situations the assessing physician may have a duty to report the IME findings to the authorities. Where there are threats uttered against any third party, a duty to report to the appropriate authorities exists. The duty to report motor vehicle drivers that are deemed incapable of operating a vehicle depends on the jurisdiction the provider practices in. As is the case with acute intoxication as a contra-indication to driving, it should be noted that several other acute contra-indications to driving exist (CMA, 2006):

- Acute psychosis;
- Condition relapses sufficient to impair perceptions, mood, or thinking;
- Medication with potentially sedating effects initiated or dose increases;
- Lack of insight or lack of cooperation with treatment;
- Lack of compliance with any conditional licensing limitations imposed by the authority;
- Suicidal plan involving crashing a vehicle;
- The intent to use a vehicle to harm others.

7.5 The nature independent assessment

The aim of the independent psychiatric evaluation is to reach specific and reliable answers to the questions posed by the retaining third party.

The domain of the independent assessment overlaps with the typical psychiatric assessment of adults, but differs in a number of ways. It is geared towards the resolution of a specific legal, administrative, or other nonclinical questions, and the respondent is not the physician's patient, and there does not exist any past or future prospects for the establishment of a patient-physician relationship. The independent assessment relies on previous or current medical records, additional documentation pertaining to the respondent's occupational circumstances, performance in the workplace, and knowledge of the existence of any workplace issues, taking into account the potential biases that may exist. In the context of an evaluation, the main focus is the collection of sufficient information to be able to provide a valid and reliable independent opinion, and the usual task of establishing a working relationship with the patient is completely avoided.

It is deemed unethical to use psychotherapeutic techniques or approaches (e.g. specialized cognitive, coercive, contingency, or motivational enhancement) to obtain information the respondent would not otherwise have offered, or to attempt to obtain information by implying or suggesting any future therapeutic involvement. The independent evaluation is by definition not an emergency evaluation, and the assessor should exercise great caution when a request is made for an emergency independent assessment. The IME is typically a time-intensive exercise, conducted over consecutive hours, the duration of which is dependent on the complexity of the case.

Although there has not been established a traditional physician-patient relationship, the IME may yield information pertaining to threats to the safety of others. Although emergency issues are relatively rare in the context of IME's, the duty of the assessing psychiatrist would be to ensure the safety of the patient and others, and a duty to report may exist. When the respondent is agitated or psychotic, or if imminent risk of harm to self or others is identified, immediate steps are required to ameliorate the risk of harm. Involvement in the IME precludes active involvement in treatment, but does not negate the duty to address immediate safety issues. Depending on the duty to report impaired drivers in the particular jurisdiction, a respondent who is under the influence of a substance at the time of the IME may have to be reported to the transportation authorities or police if there is an imminent risk of impaired driving.

The psychiatric evaluation is aimed to establish whether a mental disorder or other condition is present, and the DSM IV-TR 5-Axis formulation is used to summarize the clinical picture, which may include a differential diagnosis if uncertainty exists. The assessment includes the evaluation of longer-term issues (e.g., premorbid personality issues or disorders, pre-existing psychiatric conditions or vulnerabilities) that may impact on the outcome of the disability assessment.

7.6 The domains of the psychiatric evaluation

The independent psychiatric evaluation involves the systematic consideration of the broad domains, including:

i.   Reason for the assessment.
ii. History of the present illness.
iii. Occupational history, including exploration of workplace issues.
iv. Past psychiatric history, previous psychiatric hospitalizations, previous suicide attempts or treatment.
v.   Past and current medical history.
vi. Medication, including dosage and duration of use, as well as previous trials of use of medication, including over-the-counter preparations.
vii. Legal history, including current or past involvement, and the existence of outstanding charges.
viii. Family history.
ix. Substance-related history including (but not limited to) alcohol, caffeine, nicotine, marijuana, cocaine, opiates, sedative-hypnotic agents, stimulants, solvents, MDMA, androgenic steroids, and hallucinogens; or any combination thereof.

x. Developmental, social and interpersonal, cultural, and military history.

xi. Review of systems, to identify symptoms not already listed to date in the assessment.

xii. Functional assessment, e.g. activities of daily living (ADL), activities necessary for public transportation, Activities of Daily Living Commonly Measured in Activities of Daily Living (ADL) and Instrumental Activities of Daily Living (IADL). These include (Cocchiarella & Andersson, 2001):

Self-care, personal hygiene	Urinating, defecating, brushing teeth, combing hair, bathing, dressing oneself, eating.
Communication	Writing, typing, keyboarding, seeing, hearing, speaking, reading.
Physical activity	Standing, sitting, reclining, walking, climbing stairs.
Sensory function	Hearing, seeing, tactile feeling, tasting, smelling.
Non-specialized hand activities	Grasping, lifting, tactile discrimination.
Travel	Riding, driving, flying.
Sexual function	Orgasm, ejaculation, lubrication, erection.
Sleep	Restful, nocturnal sleep pattern.

xiii. Mental Status Examination (MSE), a systematic collection of information, is designed to obtain evidence of the existence of any mental disorder, and to augment the assessment of risk, capacity, and tolerance. In documenting the findings of the mental status examination, it is often useful to include examples illustrative of the clinical observations. The typical MSE includes the domains of (1) Appearance and general behavior. (2) Psychomotor activity, (3) Characteristics of speech, (4) Mood and affect. (4) Thought processes, (5) Thought content, (6) Perceptual disturbances, (7) Sensorium and cognition, which includes include orientation (e.g., person, place, time, situation), attention and concentration, memory (e.g., registration, short-term, long-term), and the respondent's fund of knowledge. Additional comments pertaining to intelligence, language functions (e.g., naming, comprehension, repetition, reading, writing), drawing (e.g., copying a figure or drawing a clock face), abstract reasoning (e.g., explaining similarities or interpreting proverbs), and executive functions (e.g., list making, inhibiting impulsive answers, resisting distraction, recognizing contradictions) are useful in formulating the opinion; (8) Insight; and (9) Judgment. The MSE should also include statements about the respondent's reliability as a historian. The MSE should contain documented information on the putative presence of any imminent or substantial risk of harm to self or to others.

xiv. Physical examination, if deemed contributory.

xv. Further diagnostic testing.

7.7 Assessment of work functions

To describe the dimension of putative impairment of work functioning, the assessing psychiatrist attempts to determine the potential impact the specific symptom (associated with the diagnosed mental disorder), or other reported symptoms or signs, may have on the specific work functioning. Three domains for such have been identified (Gold & Shuman, 2009):

a. Social / emotional
   - Giving directions
   - Requesting clarification
   - Initiating interpersonal contact
   - Asking for feedback on job performance
   - Responding appropriately to negative feedback
   - Initiating corrective action
   - Providing explanations
   - Describing events
   - Communicating intelligibly, fluently, coherently
   - Responding appropriately to supervision
   - Maintaining relationships with supervisors
   - Responding appropriately to supervisors
   - Responding appropriately to coworkers
   - Adapting to a new supervisor or new coworkers

b. Cognitive
   - Understanding, remembering, carrying out directions
   - Assessing own performance
   - Making decisions
   - Seeking information when necessary
   - Exercising judgment
   - Problem-solving capacity:
     - Managing multiple pressures or stresses
     - Balancing work and home life
     - Solving routine problems that make it possible to work, such as getting up on time, taking public transportation.
   - Recognizing when to stop doing one task and move on to another
   - Learning new tasks
   - Transferring learning
   - Adapting to a change in work assignment
   - Focusing on multiple tasks simultaneously
   - Screening out environmental stimuli
   - Processing information (e.g. understanding, analyzing, synthesizing)
   - Maintaining boundaries of responsibility

c. Physical
   - Maintaining fixed work schedule, including:
     - Need for flexible schedule or breaks or modified hours due to the impairment;
     - The effects of medication;
     - The need for appointments to receive treatment;
     - The need for leave to receive acute treatment.
   - Maintaining work pace
   - Maintaining stamina throughout the day

The AMA Guide to the Evaluation of Work Ability and Return to Work (AMA, 2011) suggests screening tests for establishing functional capacity. These include (adapted) the "Grocery Store" test question [*"If the individual owned his/her own grocery store, would he or she be able to find a way to work safely? If the answer is yes, then an absence from work is probably not medically required"*]. This suggests that a non-medical aspect (or psychosocial issue), as opposed to the medical condition, is creating the disability. Another test is that of the "Molehill Sign": [*"Is the individual making a mountain out of a molehill, or is an apparently minor health condition having a major effect on the individual's daily life and functions?"* In the case of an affirmative response, the issue creating disability relates to motivation, i.e. tolerance. A final test is that of "The Obstacle". The question is posed what the specific obstacle is that is preventing the individual from working *today*, hence attempting to uncover the situational or environmental obstacles to returning to work (AMA, 2011).

7.8 Documenting the results of the Independent Medical (Psychiatric and Addictions) Evaluation (IME)

Upon completion of the IME, the assessing physician should be able to respond to the questions posed. The report should restrict its scope to such questions posed, and inclusion of unnecessary information not pertinent to issues under discussion should be avoided in the interest of privacy. The IME report aims to provide a succinct overview of issues related to:

1. The DSM IV-TR diagnostic formulation and the symptoms and evidence to support such.
2. The existence of any risk issues.
3. The respondent's capacity in the context of activities of daily living, and activities outside the workplace.
4. The existence of any workplace issues.
5. Tolerance and fitness to return to work, as well as in which capacity that would be feasible.
6. Potential recommendations for further management.

Like in clinical practice, if a specific finding or item is not documented, it is reasonable to suggest that it was not tested. The source file (i.e. the notes made during the actual assessment) may be requested by the retaining third party, or in tort cases by the opposing counsel. These should be available and released only with the appropriate level of consent. Handwriting should be legible and the content should be consistent with the opinions provided and conclusions offered in the final report. The industry standards for turn-around (i.e. from assessment to report submission) are approximately ten days for IME's, and no draft versions are offered for review to the retaining party. Reports are offered in its entirety and should not be severed as this may distort the collective opinion and conclusions.

7.9 Psychiatric disorders and shift work

It is not uncommon for workers to request to be excused from shiftwork. There exist very few indications for legitimately recommending the avoidance of shift work. Under circumstances where Bipolar Disorder has been diagnosed, where unnecessary sleep disturbance or deprivation may trigger a manic episode, the worker may be restricted from conducting shift (night or rotating) work. For the majority of cases of psychiatric disorders, there is no basis for restricting shift work. Pregnancy, in the absence of another basis for imposing a restriction, is not just cause for recommending the avoidance of shift work.

7.10 The issue of over exaggeration of symptoms

Cognitive deficits resulting in erroneous comprehension, recall, and expression may lead to inaccurate reporting of information. However, there is also a real risk of malingering and deception in symptom reporting. In the absence of objective and validated correlates for most mental disorders, the assessing psychiatrist should maintain a high index of suspicion with regards to the over-exaggeration of symptoms. Exaggeration of cognitive symptoms is widespread in disability-related evaluations, and it is unwise to accept self-reported memory complaints at face value (Richman, et al., 2006). Symptom exaggeration can create a seriously misleading impression of impairment and disability, but there exists no simple measure to detect malingering during independent evaluations.

7.11 Offering a disclaimer to the IME

The IME should include offering a verbal disclaimer to the worker who is about to be assessed, but such disclaimer should also be included in the written report. This allows for sufficient protection of the assessing party and also decreases the likelihood of a future successful suit against the psychiatrist. An example of a disclaimer is as follows:

"The writer of this report is responsible for the documented comments based on reviewing the listed information, and is independent from the adjudication of claims by the requesting third party. The writer was not in a position to objectively verify the historical accuracy of all of the information provided, and if significantly inaccurate or incomplete, it may understandably impact on the accuracy of the opinions provided, and the writer's stated opinion may be subject to modification or change. The writer reserves the right to alter his opinion should further information come to light, which would warrant reconsideration of the opinion. The opinions are provided with a reasonable degree of medical certainty, and recommendations for treatment are provided independently from the requesting third party. The reader is advised to contact the writer if any clarification is required regarding the content of this report".

8. Quantifying impairment in across different classification systems and guides

The triangulation of criteria of three published rating scales (i.e. the DSM IV-TR GAF scale, the AMA Class of Impairment, and the Washington State WAC Permanent Impairments of Mental Health) describes a practical strategy to allow for quantitative objectivity in measurement of impairment, and the GAF scores have been matched through triangulation with the Washington State WAC Permanent Impairment of Mental Health (omitted from the table below), and the class of impairment of the AMA Guidelines (Williams, 2010).

In an attempt to construct a similar grid that would be applicable to the Worker's Compensation Board's definition in the authors' jurisdiction, the authors compared the AMA classes with the Alberta WCB classes of impairment (WCB, 2001).

To allow for reconciliation of the GAF scores and the rating of permanent impairment in Alberta (WCB, 2006), the authors propose the following alignment between existing practice in the jurisdiction of Alberta, Canada's WCB Permanent Impairment Rating and the DSM

IV-TR GAF scores. The alignment, although less intuitive than what has been achieved with the AMA classes of impairment, appear to offer some additional clarity in quantifying the levels of impairment through triangulation. These correlations are based on face value, best matching of the GAF score descriptors with the category in the Alberta WCB description, based severity of impairment. The impairment classes based on WCB descriptions were tentatively placed in the categories as outlined in the table below. The local jurisdiction's class I and II appear to be consistent with a GAF of 80-100, which appears dissimilar to the AMA impairment rating, and for Class V, the GAF scores from 0-20 and 21-40 appear to match. This triangulation requires further study and validation.

DSM IV-TR GAF Score	Class of Impairment (AMA, 2011)	Description of Class
80-100	1 No Impairment	No impairment detected
61-80	2 Mild Impairment	Impairment levels are compatible with most useful functioning
41-60	3 Moderate Impairment	Impairment levels are compatible with some but not all useful functioning
21-40	4 Marked Impairment	Impairment levels significantly impede useful functioning
1-20	5 Extreme Impairment	Impairment levels preclude useful functioning

Table 2.

DSM IV-TR GAF Scale (APA, 2000)	Class of Impairment: WCB Guide (WCB, 2006)	Description (WCB, 2006)
GAF 81-100: - Superior functioning in a wide range of activities, life's problems never seem to get out of hand, is sought out by others because of his or her many positive qualities. No symptoms.	Class I: No impairment, 0%	The worker: - Is able to carry on with all the activities of daily living; and - Is able to perform work related duties without difficulty under normal conditions of stress, or - May exhibit intermittent pain behavior without restriction of functional ability.
- Absent or minimal symptoms, good functioning in all areas, interested and involved in a wide variety of activities, socially effective, generally satisfied with life, no more than everyday problems or concerns.	Class II: Minimal impairment 1-10%	The worker: - Is able to carry out all the activities of daily living with some decrease in personal and social efficiency, AND - exhibits mild anxiety in the form of restlessness, uneasiness and tension which result in minimal functional limitation, OR - exhibits pain behavior causing a minimal restriction of functional

DSM IV-TR GAF Scale (APA, 2000)	Class of Impairment: WCB Guide (WCB, 2006)	Description (WCB, 2006)
		ability, AND - is able to function in most vocational settings but develops secondary psychogenic symptoms under normal conditions of stress.
GAF 61-80: - If symptoms are present, they are transient and expectable reactions to psychosocial stressors; no more than slight impairment in social, occupational, or school functioning. - Some mild symptoms OR some difficulty in social, occupational, or school functioning, but generally functioning pretty well, has some meaningful interpersonal relationships.	Class III: Mild Impairment 11-30%	The worker: - is capable of taking care of all personal needs at home but may experience a reduced confidence level and an increased dependency outside the home, AND - experiences a definite limitation of personal and social efficiency, OR - suffers episodic anxiety, agitation, and unusual fear of situations which appear to threaten re-injury, OR - exhibits persistent pain behavior, associated with signs of emotional withdrawal and depression (e.g. loss of appetite, insomnia, chronic fatigue, low noise tolerance and mild psychomotor retardation), OR in the case of conversion reactions, consistently avoids the use of affected part leading to restriction of everyday activities, AND - will probably require vocational adjustment depending upon both the signs and symptoms present and the nature of the pre-accident work.
GAF 41-60: - Moderate symptoms OR moderate difficulty in social, occupational, or school functioning. - Serious symptoms OR any serious impairment in social, occupational, or school functioning.	Class IV: Moderate Impairment 31-50%	The worker: - Suffers definite deterioration of familial adjustment and incipient breakdown of social integration, AND - in the case of conversion reactions, exhibits bizarre behavior and a tendency to avoid anxiety creating situations to the point of significant restriction of everyday activities, AND - may require periodic confinement to the home or a treatment facility and will need significant vocational adjustment.
GAF 21-40: - Some impairment in reality testing or communication,	Class V: Severe Impairment 51-75%	The worker: - exhibits a chronic and severe inability to function both in and out of

DSM IV-TR GAF Scale (APA, 2000)	Class of Impairment: WCB Guide (WCB, 2006)	Description (WCB, 2006)
OR major impairment in several areas, such as work, school, family relations, judgment, thinking, or mood. - Behavior is considerably influenced by delusions or hallucinations or serious impairment of communication or judgment OR inability to function in almost all areas.		the home, - suffers obvious loss of interest in the environment, extreme emotional irritability, emotional lability and uncontrolled outbursts of temper, OR - experiences mood changes with psychotic levels of depression, severe motor retardation and psychological regression, AND requires constant supervision and/or confinement as well as major vocational adjustment.
GAF 1-20: Some danger of hurting self or others, OR Occasionally fails to maintain minimal personal hygiene, OR Gross impairment in communication. Persistent danger of severely hurting self or others, OR Persistent inability to maintain minimal personal hygiene, OR Serious suicidal act with clear expectation of death.	**Also Class V:** Severe Impairment	**The worker (as above):** - exhibits a chronic and severe inability to function both in and out of the home, - suffers obvious loss of interest in the environment, extreme emotional irritability, emotional lability and uncontrolled outbursts of temper, OR - experiences mood changes with psychotic levels of depression, severe motor retardation and psychological regression, AND requires constant supervision and/or confinement as well as major vocational adjustment.

Table 3.

9. Providing remedies through comprehensive mental health disability management

9.1 Towards an operational definition for Mental Health Disability Management:

Mental Health Disability Management (MHDM) is a relatively new field involving a range of health professionals from different disciplines. The authors offer the formal definition of "the restoration of functional capacity, or the prevention of deterioration thereof, in a person who has been chronically or permanently impaired as a result of psychopathology, mental and/or addiction-related disorders". MHDM should be offered on the least restrictive level of care that is likely to be effective and proven to be safe, consistent with the principles of treatment matching in other areas of healthcare. It aims at developing the individual's existing resources, mobilizing additional resources, and to correct the relational interplay between impairment, the respondent, and the environment, collectively responsible for the disability. MHDM has a broad focus and is concerned with an individualized approach to limiting risk and ensuring safety, improving capacity (or preventing further deterioration), increasing tolerance, remedying negative attitudes towards MHDM, and increasing motivation to return to work.

With financial expenditure related to psychiatric disability appearing to be out of control, and the existence of an empirical body of evidence suggesting the economic advantages of management of psychiatric disability, the authors are observing a growing trend and demand for evidence-based MHDM.

9.2 The goals of MHDM

In 1981 the World Health Organization stated that the aims of rehabilitation should be to reduce the impact of disabling conditions and identified three levels of action to bring this about. These same three goals (Harder and Scott, 2005) translate into the goals of MHDM:

- Reducing the occurrence of impairments
- Limiting or reversing disability caused by impairment
- Preventing the transition of disability to *handicap* (which is defined as a disadvantage for a given individual, resulting from an impairment or disability, which limits or prevents the fulfillment of a role that is normal for the individual).

9.3 The components of MHDM

MHDM includes a variety of components: prevention (primary), assessment, claim management (secondary, tertiary prevention), accommodation, return to work, and aftercare monitoring. Early identification and intervention are superior to lengthy and delayed protocols of assessment and management. Identification of mental health impairment and disability is a shared responsibility between employer and employee, and the responsibility of co-workers to report safety concerns or impairment in co-workers is beneficial in early initiation of remedies to prevent injuries and disability.

- Under ideal circumstances, workplace mental health promotion programs have the potential to prevent the development of a range of disorders. These prevent the development of mental disorders and addiction in vulnerable individuals and allow for prevention of update of drugs to cope or to self-medicate subjective distress.
- When a safety issue or a performance deficit has been identified, and there is reasonable suspicion of the existence of psychopathology, a mental disorder, or risky behavior, the confidential collection of accurate information pertaining to the health status of the respondent is mandated. The minimum data set in this regard should include an objective diagnosis (if any), formulated in a 5-Axis format, which includes a Global Assessment of Functioning, information pertaining to the safety issue / performance deficit that brought the case to the attention, information on putative predisposing, precipitating, and modulating factors in this regard, as well as the existence of any workplace issues. The claimant's motivation to return to work and the factors that could be affecting it should be assessed, and routine screening for any substance-related disorder or issues, which may be impacting the employee's presentation and recovery, should be explored. The symptoms reported by the employee should be documented, along with their frequency, severity, and duration, and the objective clinical findings during the examination, including the results of any mental status testing, should be included. A determination should be made whether the objective findings are consistent with

the subjectively reported findings, and if there is any evidence of malingering, symptom amplification, or simulation.

A routine part of the independent evaluation should include the previous psychiatric history, including previous hospitalizations, previous suicide attempts, and previous psychiatric treatment received. The assessment should include questions pertaining to adherence to previous treatment, as well as the nature of any trials offered, e.g. the dose and duration of pharmacotherapy. If counseling or psychotherapy were offered in the past, a determination should be made if this represented a reasonable and appropriately focused trial, and if a reasonable level of adherence was achieved. With an appropriate description of previous and current treatment modalities, the employee's response to treatment should also be determined, along with the identification of factors that might have impacted on the clinical course and recovery.

• In all cases the existence of personality disorders or the prominent use of specific ego defense mechanisms should be assessed, to determine if any DSM IV-TR Axis II factors are impacting on the response to treatment? Activities of daily living, such as household chores, child care, hobbies, interests, ability to socialize or travel, and any academic or vocational pursuits should be assessed and reported on.

With the completion of a standardized and comprehensive psychiatric assessment, an opinion can be rendered pertaining to risk, tolerance, and capacity. To offer informed opinions pertaining to any putative restrictions and limitations, which may exist, the assessor should obtain sufficient information regarding the essential duties of the job, any potentially safety-sensitive elements of the job, and of any potential workplace issues the employee may not have reported.

Following the completion of the comprehensive psychiatric assessment, discussion should ensue with the employer to assist in informing further MHDM.

9.5 Claim management

This component falls outside the scope of practice of the assessing physician, and it is recommended that the assessing physician clearly communicate the boundaries. The reporting on impairment, psychiatric illness, capacity, risk, and tolerance are not implied to construe a recommendation pertaining to the adjudication of any claims or legal matters. The opinions provided also do not suggest that a specific administrative function be made or enforced, and are offered independently from the requesting party's interests. Many persons becoming ill, psychiatrically or otherwise, find it challenging to navigate the maize of healthcare systems. It falls outside the scope of the physician conducting the assessment to assist in such navigation as it might be interpreted (by the worker undergoing the assessment) as the establishment of a physician-patient relationship. Such relationship would be associated with other duties and obligations. At a time with the worker is psychiatrically unwell; he/she may be particularly vulnerable, and less inclined to assume responsibility for accessing care unless additional support is offered.

9.6 The Duty to Accommodate

Under Human Rights legislation, the employer has a duty to accommodate disability to the point of undue hardship. This is a legal determination, falling outside the scope of this manuscript.

9.7 Return-to-work

The safe and timely return to work has favorable human and financial results (Curtis & Scott, 2004), and is often therapeutic in psychiatric conditions. Lengthy disability decreases the likelihood of a return to work.

9.8 Follow-up monitoring

Following the establishment of a diagnosis and after furnishing treatment recommendations, the worker should be matched with the appropriate level of evidence-based treatment interventions. In cases where a substance-related disorder was diagnosed, the need for ongoing random drug screening may be necessary, within what is permissible under human rights or disability legislation.

10. Avoiding common pitfalls in the assessment and management of mental health disability

The authors offer a non-exhaustive table of 10 common pitfalls (along with proposed solutions) in the practice of conducting psychiatric IME's:

Description of common pitfall:	Proposed remedy:
1. Dual agency conflicts.	Treating physicians should avoid involvement in offering conclusions pertaining to forensic matters. Similarly, physicians conducting IMEs should not become involved in treatment, in the context of a traditional physician-patient relationship. The assessing physician should refrain from acting as an advocate for the worker, but is also not an advocate for the retaining party.
2. Equating mental disorder diagnosis with impairment and disability.	There is a non-linear relationship between mental disorder, impairment, and disability. Rigorous and distinction between these matters is required, and each domain should be quantified based on collected evidence. Assessment of disability should be related to work-specific functions. The criteria for disability are determined by the particular third party and may vary across jurisdictions. The Social Security Administration's Criteria for Total disability requires that the mental disorder persist despite adequate treatment, for at least 12 months, at a level that produces at least two of the following: 1. Marked restriction in ADL; 2. Marked difficulties in maintaining social functioning; 3. Marked difficulties in maintaining concentration, persistence, or pace, and 4. Repeated episodes of decompensation, each of

	extended duration.
3. Assumption that occupation is an automatic and causal factor in mental disorders.	Work is therapeutic and is rarely considered causally related to the development of mental disorders. Consideration should be given to workplace issues, motivation, psychosocial issues, and other non-occupational factors in determining causality.
4. Reporting without the use of standardized diagnostic language, e.g. using "depression" to describe a Major Depressive Disorder.	Strict adherence to the diagnostic classification system of choice, e.g. the DSM IV-TR or the ICD-10.
5. Reliance on Mental Status Examination and GAF scores alone to determine degree of impairment.	The systematic determination of functioning should be conducted.
6. Failure to obtain valid consent.	Consent should be informed and valid, and this task should not be delegated to administrative personnel. The explanation of the scope and nature of the assessment should be the duty of the assessing physician, and should include the opportunity for the worker to ask questions.
7. Failure to report imminent risk of harm.	In a small number of situations there may exist a duty to report imminent risk of harm to self or others, or a reporting to the appropriate transportation authorities.
8. Failure to take Axis II conditions into consideration	A standard IME should include an opinion pertaining to the presence of any possible Personality Disorder, or the salient use of defense mechanisms that may impact on the individual's clinical condition.
9. Reliance on self-reporting only in the context of symptoms, e.g. cognitive symptoms.	The assessing physician should take into account that cognitive dysfunction cannot be determined by relying on self-report only. Exaggeration in this context is widespread, and objective measures are required to validate the presence of any cognitive disturbance.
10. Failure to provide a well-substantiated report, or failure to respond to the referral source's questions.	Care should be taken to ensure that the questions posed to the assessing physician are clarified in advance of conducting the assessment, and the report should focus on responding to these questions only. If an opinion is reached based on the review of records only, such fact should be clearly communicated in the report.

Table 4.

11. Summary

Disability is on the increase, and mental disorders are projected to be the leading cause of disability in future. Work is therapeutic, and most individuals do not experience an exacerbation of mental disorders as a result of working.

Conducting independent occupational assessments to determine capacity, risk, tolerance and fitness for work, is a specialized area of psychiatry, with its own pitfalls and caveats. Many psychiatrists experience this as intrusive and feel they are ill-prepared to navigate this arena.

This chapter outlined the common mental disorders, encountered in clinical and occupational settings, including Depressive Disorders, Anxiety Disorders, Substance-Related Disorders, and Personality Disorders. Of central importance is the duty to objectively measure impairment, and to not only rely on the diagnosis to determine the level of impairment. The non-linear relationship between mental disorder, impairment and disability is a key concept, and utilizing a template for conducting independent assessments may assist in bypassing some of the most common pitfalls.

The assessment of the functional impairment is the first step towards implementing the appropriate level of mental health disability management. The enjoyment of the human right to optimal health, without discrimination on the grounds of any disability, is vital to a person's well-being.

12. References

Armstrong, J. (2008). A Business Case for Conversations on Mental Health. Canadian Mental Health Association, Calgary Region. Available at:
http://www.cmha.calgary.ab.ca/copernicus/The%20Business%20Case%20for%20 Web%20link.pdf

Aneshensel, C.S., & Phelan, J.C. (Eds.) (1999). *Handbook of the Sociology of Mental Health*, Kluwer Academic Publishers, ISBN 9780387325163 , New York

American Medical Association. Guides to the Evaluation of Permanent Impairment. Chicago, IL: AMA Press; 2001:1-613

American Psychiatric Association (2000) Diagnostic and Statistical Manual of Mental Disorders, 4th Edition, text-revised. American Psychiatric Association. ISBN 9780890420256. Arlington VA

Blustein, D.L. (2008). The Role of Work in Psychological Health and Well-being: A Conceptual, Historical, and Public Policy Perspective. *American Psychologist.* 63(4):228-240

Bonnie, R.J. (Ed). (1997). Mental Disorder, Work Disability and the Law. University of Chicago Press, ISBN 9780226064505, Chicago

Canadian Medical Association (2006). *Determining medical fitness to operate motor vehicles. CMA driver's guide.* 7th ed. Ottawa (ON): The Association. Available at:
http://www.cma.ca/index.php/ci_id/18223/la_id/1.htm

Cocchiarella, L & Anderson, GBJ, eds. (2001). *Guides to the Evaluation of Permanent Impairment.* 5th ed., American Medical Association. Chicago

Curtis, J., & Scott L. (2004). Integrating disability management into strategic plans. *American Association of Occupational Health Nurses Journal.* 52(7):298-301

Dewa, C., Lesage, A., Goering, P., Caveen, M. (2004). Nature and prevalence of mental illness in the workplace. *Healthcare Papers.* 5(2): 12-29

Don, A.S., & Carragee, E.J. (2009) Is the self-reported history accurate in patients with persistent axial pain after a motor vehicle accident? *Spine J.* 9:4-12

Engel, G.L. (1977). The Need for a New Medical Model: a Challenge for Biomedicine. *Science*, 196, 129-136

Greenberg, S.A., & Shuman, D.W. (1997). Irreconcilable conflict between therapeutic and forensic rules. *Professional Psychology Research and Practice.* 28:50-57

Gold, L.H., & Shuman, D.W. (2009). Evaluating Mental Health Disability in the Workplace – Model, Process, and Analysis. Springer. ISBN: 9781441901521. New York.

Harder, H.G., & Scott, L.R. (2005). Comprehensive Disability Management. Elsevier Churchill Livingstone, ISBN 0443101132, London

Kessler, R.C., Berglund, P., Demler, O., et al. (2005). Lifetime prevalence and age-of-onset distributions of DSM-IV in the National Comorbidity Survey Replication. *Archives of General Psychiatry*, 62, 593-602

Kessler, R.C., Chiu, W.T., Demler, O., & Walters, E.E. (2005). Prevalence, severity, and comorbidity of the 12-month DSM-IV disorders in the National Comorbidity Survey Replication. *Archives of General Psychiatry*, 62, 617-627

O'Toole, J. (1982) Work and love (mostly work). *Journal of Psychiatric Treatment and Evaluation.* 4,227-237.

Richman, J., Green, P., Gervais, R., et al. (2006). Objective Tests of Symptom Exaggeration in Independent Medical Examinations. *Journal of Occupational and Environmental Medicine.* 48;3:303-311.

Stephens, T., Joubert, N. Health Canada. Population and public health branch (2001). The economic burden of mental health problems in Canada. *Chronic disease in Canada*; 22 (1).

Talmage, J.B., Melhorn J.M., Hyman M.H. (2011). *AMA Guides to the Evaluation of Work Ability and Return to Work, 2nd Edition* American Medical Association, ISBN 9871603595308, Chicago

Thomas, J.C., & Hersen, M. (2004). Psychopathology in the Workplace. Brunner-Routledge, ISBN 9780415933797, New York

Wang, P., Simon, G., Kessler, R. (2003). The economic burden of depression and the cost-effectiveness of treatment. *The International Journal of Methods in Psychiatric Research.* 12(1):22-33.

Watson Wyatt Worldwide. (2005). Staying at work: Making the connection to a healthy organization. United States: Watson Wyatt Worldwide. Available at: http://www.towerswatson.com/

Watson Wyatt Worldwide. (2007). Staying at Work: Effective presence at work.2007 Survey report. Canada: Watson Wyatt Worldwide. Available at: http://www.towerswatson.com/

Williams, C.D. (2010) Disability and Occupational Assessment: Objective Diagnosis and Quantitative Impairment Rating. *Harvard Review of Psychiatry.* 18:336-352.

Workers' Compensation Board Alberta. Alberta Permanent Clinical Impairment Guide (2006). Available at http://www.wcb.ab.ca/pdfs/public/policy/manual/a_d.pdf

World Medical Association Statement on Patient Advocacy and Confidentiality, (2006). Available at: http://www.wma.net/en/30publications/10policies/a11/

Part 2

Control

5

Early Intervention in Psychiatry Challenges & Opportunities

Mamdouh El-Adl
Queen University, Kingston, Ontario
Canada

1. Introduction

We may agree that psychiatry has advanced so much within a relatively short life span. Civilized life is a sign & reason for good physical and mental health. Herodotus in V Century BC expressed his admiration for the health of Egyptians, saying that they were the healthiest in the world, that "Egyptian are different from other people… they take their meals outside their homes, while they attend to their needs inside". Diodorus Siculus in the first Century BC stated that" the whole manner of life of the Egyptians was so wholesome that it would appear as though it had been arranged according to the rules of a learned physician rather than those of the legislator (Ghaliongui 1983).

Legislation may have an important role to play at some stage of nation's building, but with progress of life, maturity and stability of the population the legislation may be of less importance than previously.

The first mental hospital in the world was built Ephesus of the old Roman empire in the ancient times. In Middle ages there was a mental hospital in Baghdad, Iraq in 705 AD. This was followed by hospitals in Cairo (800 AD0, Damascus 1270 Adand Aleppo in Syria). At the at time, mentally ill patients were being burnt, condemend and punished in Europe (Okasha, 1993)

Psychiatric asylums were landmarks in the history of psychiatric care. Mental Asylums were essentially to help 2 main purposes:

1. Caring for & protecting the mentally ill people
2. Public protection.

In 18th Century some documentation in the Journal of the Liverpool Psychiatric Club may demonstrate how psychiatry was at that time (Fig 1,2) (Psychiatry in Liverpool,1800).

1.1 Early attempts to understand mental illness

In a great step forwards, Benjamin Rush invented a tranquilizer chair as he believed that mental illness is due to irritation of blood vessels in the brain and his treatment method included bleeding, purging, hot & cold baths and mercury and he invented a tranquilizer chair (Fig4).

This style of thinking is not considered to be scientifically based or evidence based by the rules of our time nowadays but was a very courageous attempt to understand more about mental illness at this relatively early time. With this development the beginning of thinking about mental illness, its underlying causes and how to treat started. This may have been an early attempt in the wrong direction but we may agree that lot of discoveries in the field of medicine were not well-planned or evidence –based but started as trial & error. Most of our recent styles of thinking in the era of evidence-based medicine are relatively new. However there was a believe that Evidence-based medicine, whose philosophical origins extend back to mid-19th century. Earlier, is the conscientious, explicit and judicious use of current best evidence in making decisions about the care of individual patients? The practice of evidence-based medicine means integrating individual clinical expertise with the best available external clinical evidence from systematic research. By individual clinical expertise we mean the proficiency and judgment that we individual clinicians acquire through clinical experience and clinical practice (Sackett, 2006)

Liverpool, 18th century: Dealing with Mentally Ill in Liverpool in The 18th Century

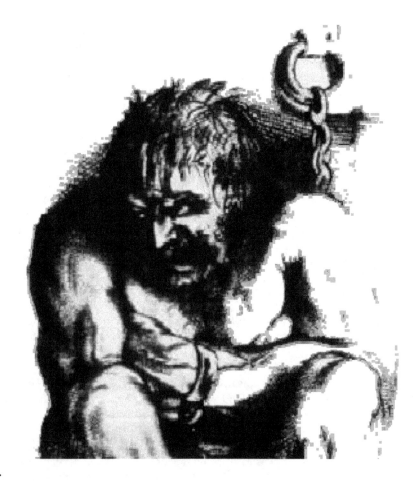

Fig. 1.

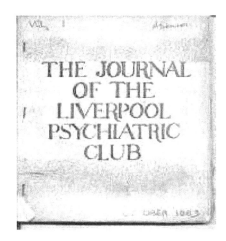

Fig. 2.

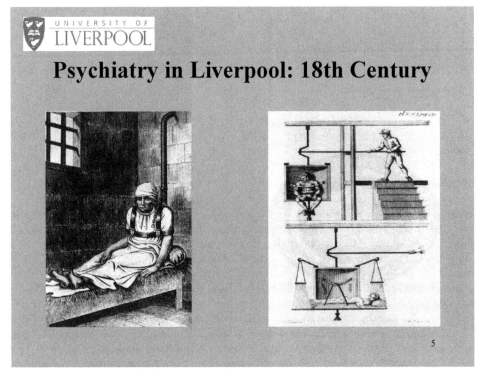

Fig. 3. Care for the mentally ill in Liverpool in the 18th century[3]

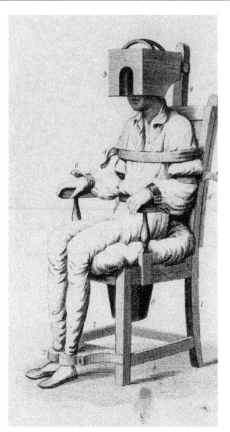

Fig. 4. Tranquilizing chair[4]

However, with further development, Modern psychiatric hospitals evolved from, and eventually replaced the older lunatic asylums.

1.2 The discovery of chlorpromazine
The discovery of phenothiazines, the first family of antipsychotic agents has its origin in the development German dye industry, at the end of the 19th century (Graebe, Liebermann, Bernthsen). Up to 1940 they were employed as antiseptics, antihelminthics and antimalarials (Ehrlich, Schulemann, Gilman). Finally, in the context of research on antihistaminic substances in France after World War II (Bovet, Halpern, Ducrot) the chlorpromazine was synthesized at Rhône-Poulenc Laboratories (Charpentier, Courvoisier, Koetschet) in December 1950. Its introduction in anaesthesiology, in the antishock area (lytic cocktails) and "artificial hibernation" techniques, is reviewed (Laborit), and its further psychiatric clinical introduction in 1952, with initial discrepancies between the Parisian Val-de-Grâce (Laborit, Hamon, Paraire) and Sainte-Anne (Delay, Deniker) hospital groups. The first North-American publications on the introduction of chlorpromazine took place in 1954 (Lehmann, Winkelman, Bower). The introduction of chlorpromazine in the USA was more difficult due to their strong psychoanalytic tradition. The consolidation of the neuroleptic

therapy took place in 1955, thanks to a series of scientific events, which confirmed the antipsychotic efficacy of the chlorpromazine. (Lopez-Munoz et al 2005)

1.3 Closure of mental asylums & the beginning of psychiatric units attached to general hospitals

The development of the modern psychiatric hospital is also the story of the rise of organised, institutional psychiatry. While there were earlier institutions that housed the 'insane' the arrival of institutionalisation as a solution to the problem of madness was very much an event of the nineteenth century. To illustrate this with one regional example, in England at the beginning of the nineteenth century there were, perhaps, a few thousand 'lunatics' housed in a variety of disparate institutions but by 1900 that figure had grown to about 100,000. That this growth coincided with the growth of madness, later known as psychiatry, as a medical specialism is not coincidental.

The treatment of inmates in early lunatic asylums was sometimes brutal and focused on containment and restraint. With successive waves of reform, development and the introduction of effective evidence-based treatments, modern psychiatric hospitals provide a primary emphasis on treatment, and attempt where possible to help patients control their own lives in the outside world.

Closure of Mental Asylums & re-integration of people diagnosed with mental illness was claimed by some to have been associated with increased violence in the community. This matter was considered to be an important point to de discussed or even studied. Research did not confirm that release of mentally ill individuals or what was called at that time care in the community was a reason for increased violence and crimes in the community. Some research and published papers addressed this possibility and concluded that mental illness as a single factor may not be responsible for this (Ian Kooyman et al, 2007) and some schoolars called fortigtening and improving mental health legislations to minimise the possibility of loss to care (falling off the net) like Care Programme Approach (CPA) after certain famous cases e.g. happened in the UK e.g. Christopher Clunis and murdering Jonathan Zito. After a big famous investigation they concluded that everybody was to be blamed psychiatrists, social workers, the police, community psychiatric nurses, the Crown Prosecution Service, the probation service, hostel staff, and private sector care workers. (Timmins, 1994).

The use of a combination of psychiatric drugs and Psychotherapy. These treatments can be involuntary under the power of the Mental Health Act which gives the psychiatrists the power to treat even if refused by the patient in many countries. These powers were questioned by the Anti-Psychiatric movement and human rights activists.

1.4 Community Treatment Order (CTO)

More recently in countries like UK the Mental Health Act (The Mental Health Act 2005) has been updated giving some powers to enforce treatment in the community "Community Treatment Order" (CTO). However some viewed these as insufficient changes & some human rights activists viewed these as violations of human rights.

The CTO was considered by many mental health specialists as a good step forward towards ensuring that treatment can access people diagnosed with mental illness and refuse treatment while in the community. However the law has not been able to please everybody, on one hand most mental health professionals perceive it as not enough while human right activists view it as a sort of violation of human rights. An important notice that Mental health Professionals had found initially CTO in UK of limited benefit which may reflect more about the understanding & use of the new Mental Health Act. However, the initial impression of CTO that has been used for sometime in North America especially Ontario Canada seem to be more positive. This may need to be researched and learning from the experience of use across the Atlantic to learn from each other's experience.

1.5 Mental Health Act

It is important to remember that there are some varrying number of countries across the world of varying % that have no Mental Health Act which may be attributed to different factors. These countries may include % in Africa, Asia & east meditrranean & countries in America, (Wikipedia, 2007). With the improved awareness of human rights, the numbers of countries that have a Mental Health Act will hopefully gradually increase to include all patients on the earth. It is hoped that with the continuous efforts of World Psychiatric Association (WPA) and other relevant organisations e.g. WHO more countries will have its own Mental Health Act that would suit its culture and protect patients' rights.

Regions	With legislation	No legislation
Africa	59%	41%
The Americas	73%	27%
Eastern Mediterranean	59%	41%
Europe	96%	4%
South-East Asia	67%	33%
Western Pacific	72%	28%

Table 1. % of countries all over the world regions with or without Mental Health Act

Most psychiatric hospitals now restrict any device that can take photos and aim to protect patients dignity & human rights.

1.6 Electroconvulsive therapy (ECT)

Elelectroconvulsive Therapy (Previously known as Electeric Shock) was first introduced in 1938 by Italian neuropsychiatrists Ugo Celettis and Lucio Bini gained widespread use as a form of treatment in the 1940s and 1950s.

This Treatment Modality has been successfully used as therapy for mental illness for about 80 years. It may have been subject to various improvements but the original principle remains the same. It is considered to a relatively one of the safest & effective types of therapy. ECT remains the most effective treatment for major depression and a rapidly effective treatment for life- threatening psychiatric conditions, unlike conteporaneous somatic therapies, ECT remains in the active treatment portfolio of modern therapeutics.

It is estimated that approximately 100,000 patients have received ECT annuallyin the USA. A limiting Factor in its use has been the adverse effects of confusion and memory loss associated with associated with the course of treatment. However major innovation in ECT technique to diminish cognitive effects while maintaining benefits. New development in ECT techniques over offer the hope that this form of treatment will find better acceptance among psychiatrists and patients (Kaplan & Sadock, 2007).

The developments did not stop at the improvements of hospitals & hospital care or the community but included advances in drug development. Antipsychotics developed into Atypical Antipsychotics with less side effects and more safety if taken in overdose. However one major problem raised concern which is tendency of the new Antipsychotics to induce weight gain with varriable degrees and sometimes accused of precipitating Diabetes Mellitus.

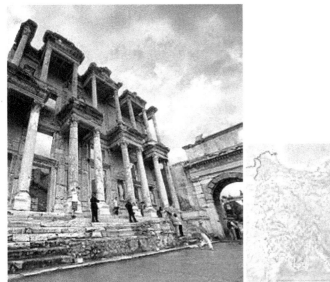
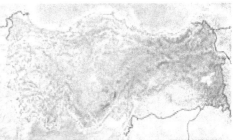

Ephesus: The ancient Roman City (Located in Turkey as per map)

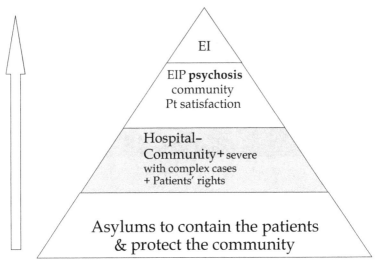

EI: early intervention, EIP: early Intervention in Psychosis,

Fig. 3. History of Psychiatry is developing relatively with a good momentum[5]

2. The importance of community care

We may have different views about care in the community but there is enough evidence that care in the community has been benefitial. We agree that care in the community is not a replacement for hospital care but compliment it. Unfortunately psychiatric services & resources are not well developed to the same extent all over the world. The following story may be an example that would be an evidence for the importance of community care. A mother killed her 4 year old daughter and attempted to kill her newly born baby.

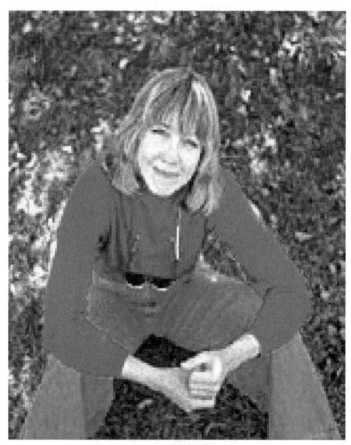

Picture picked up from the net not related to the real incidence for confidentiality.
• 23Sundayالأولى الصفحة

> اخبار الدار02:01 آخــر تحديـــث 21-03-2008 استقرار حالة الأم القاتلة والابنة الرضيعةدبي سيد الضبع: أكد الدكتور فيصل البدري رئيس قسم الجراحة بمستشفى راشد بدبي ان الحالة الصحية للأم   المتهمة بقتل ابنها البالغ من العمر 4 سنوات والشروع في قتل ابنتها الرضيعة "عامان" بعدما اصابتها بجروح بالغة أدت لتهتك الطحال والمعدة والكبد وجرح قطعي بالعمود الفقري أدى إلى تسرب سائل النخاع الشوكي مستقرة وفي حالة صحية جيدة بينما راحت تسيطر عليها حالة اكتئاب نفسي منعها من الحديث والتفاعل مع كل من يحاول الاقتراب منها وهي الحالة التي وصفها . واضاف في تصريح لـ"الخليج" ان الطفلة الرضيعة ترقد حالياً بقسم الانعاش التابع للعناية المركزة بمستشفى راشد بدبي بعد ان شهدت حالتها استقراراً نسبياً ومن المتوقع خروج الطفلة من قسم الانعاش خلال اسبوع على اقصى تقدير.ومن جهة أخرى من المنتظر أن تحال الام فور امتثالها للشفاء للنيابة العامة.

Translation of Arabic News:

A mother killed her 4 year old child, Dr Albadry, Head of Surgical Dept stated that the mother's condition is stable & her newly born baby is OK[6]. However this tells us that Psychiatric resources and services are not developed to the same extent all over the world, why? This may be related to local culture, economic factors, available resources, service priorities and service planning.

3. First episode psychosis studies

In a UK study addressed GPs experience with first episode psychosis we found out that Stigma remained a strong reason for patients and their families to refuse referral of the individual to see a psychiatrist. This could be imagined in a less developed country but not in a well developed country like UK, however, stigma of mental illness sill a strong reason to deter patients and their family members from first psychiatric referral. This supports Norman Sartorius Who stated that :"Stigma attached to mental illness is the main obstacle to the provision of mental health care[8] This may indicate the need for more work on stigma. We probably need to think of Anti-stigma Programmes not only a campaign.

It was also found that patients with first episode psychosis are less likely to ask for referral to see the psychiatrist but if offered this by their GP they are likely to accept referral. It is very important that we consider public education as a priority in our programmes worldwide. One important point that came out of this study is that GPs feel less inclined to treat psychosis in general especially early psychosis. The study did not address GPs prescribing trends in early psychosis. However GPs appear to be more comfortable treating depression than psychosis. This may be due to training programmes focusing on GPs treating depression to lower suicide rates. Does this indicate that psychosis especially early psychosis will remain the business of psychiatrists and not GPs. More importantly that early diagnosis of psychosis will need to be by specialist care not by primary care. One of the ways that can change the picture is to review GP education and training to give more attention to the area of psychosis. The answer for this question can only be answered with more time.

Interestingly in an Egyptian study on "Factors associated with delayed access to care in a rural Egyptian setting" lack of knowledge, financial factors and stigma were on the top of the list. It is obvious to us that lack of knowledge about mental illness is an important obstacle in developing & developed countries as well. In a Canadian study, treatment may be delayed if youth, young adults and parents are not aware of the early signs and symptoms of psychosis, the need for early diagnosis and treatment and where and how to get help. This article describes the use of the development of an early psychosis public education program's objectives designed to meet the learning needs of the target population (youth and young adults aged 15–30 years and their parents).

Another finding in the Egyptian Study was that DUP was about one year and this nearly the same in Studies of developed countries, this may be due to small sample studied in Egyptian study or due to presence of high% of affective psychoses in Egyptian study or this may mean that this is the natural course of the disease regardless the type of intervention or cultural difference i.e. patients with psychosis will arrive relatively late to service.

This may alert us to the need to the importance of working together to develop an international anti-stigma programme that would be culturally compatible worldwide. In the case of Egypt & culturally and economically similar countries, improving public education about mental illness and developing a viable & effective national health insurance system is likely to play an important role in health promotion in general including mental health.

In his efforts to promote early intervention in psychosis, Professor Patrick McGorie from Australia developed a Clinical staging model Framework for Psychiatric Disorders (fig. 5) that correlates clinical signs with treatment. This may put psychiatrists while handling early psychosis in line with physicians & surgeons while treating early stages of cancer (Yung & McGorry, 2007.

It is very interesting and motivating that we can see developments in psychiatry are developing with big steps to catch up with our fellows in other braches of medicine thanks to the efforts of all those who devoted their life to help their patients worldwide.

Clinical Staging Model Framework for Psychotic Disorders (Yung & McGorry, 2007)			
stage	Def.	Target Population	Potential intervention	Markers
0	-? risk of psychotic disorder - No symptoms	FD teenage Rs of probands	? MH literacy, Family+ drug edu, Cog Skills train.	SPEmovements, P50, niacin sensiti.
1a	-mild/nonspecific symptoms including neurocognitive -mild functional change or ?	-Teenagers screening -Ref by GPs & school counsellors	formal MH literacy, family psycho-education, active drug misuse? , formal CBT	Trait & state candidates where feasible
1b	Ultra high risk: moderate but subthreshold symptoms e.g. neurocognitive changes & function. changes to caseneness	Ref by GP, Education, Welfare agencies, ER	As 1a	Niacin sensitivity, folate status, MRI, HTPA axis dysregulation
2	FEPsychosis, full threshold disorder, mod.-severe symptoms, neurocog. Deficits, functional ? , (GAF: 30 – 50)	Ref by GP, Education, ER, Specialist care agencies, drug & alcohol services	As 1 + Atypical antipsychotic Vocational rehabilitation	State & trait markers & progression
3a	Incomplete remission from FEP Could be linked to stage 4	Primary & specialist services	As 2 + focus on medical & psychosocial→full Remiss	As 2
3b	Relapse/recurrence of psychosis, stabilises with treatment at a GAF level	As 3a	As 3a + emphasis on relapse prevention & early warning signs strategies	As 2
3c	Multiple relapses, impact of illness is objectively present.	Specialist service	As 3b + emphasis on long term stabilisation	As 2
4	Severe persistent or unremitting judged on symptoms, neurocognition &disability criteria	As 3c	As 3c + emphasis on Clozapine & Social participation	As 2

Fig. 5. Clinical Staging Model Framework for Psychotic Disorders (Yung & McGorry, 2007)

3.1 Challenges

1. Evidence based practice: further integration of research into clinical practice & Service planning is not always cheap but benefits are likely to outweigh costs.
2. Early intervention needs to be more inclusive e.g. Mood Disorders, Eating Disorders,....etc..
3. A preventive approach is necessary especially in Child Psychiatry
4. Stigma: we need Anti-stigma Programmes not only campaigns.

5. Third world countries patients: should not be forgotten.

3.2 Opportunities

1. Bringing Psychiatry more into medicine.
2. Further integration of Hospital care into Community programs.
3. Strengthening the Interface between secondary and primary care.

The Challenges are numerous and opportunities can be increased but we need to remain determined to make the future of Psychiatry & psychiatric patients a better future worldwide.

One important question that may need to be understood: do we expect that early intervention in psychiatry is going to be cheaper in cost compare to traditional care. The careful understanding and studying of this matter may tell us different answer that may disappoint some of us. The same may apply to working on evidence-based, is it likely to be cheaper? The experts believe that early intervention in psychiatry or working on evidence-based rules are likely to be associated with increased financial cost rather than reducing the cost. However, it may be important to do the appropriate practice with more cost than to practice inappropriately.

4. References

Crisp, pp373 – 375, published by the Royal Society of Medicine press ltd. Liverpool Psychiatric Club website accessed on 06.2011

www.uphs.upenn.edu/paharc/features/brush.html, accessed on 25.06.2011

EL-Adl M (2009) Presented at Queen University, Kingston, Ontario, Canada under the title: Early Intervention in Psychiatry

EL-Adl M, Elmahdy, M, Anis M (2008) First episode psychosis: Factors associated with delayed access to care in a rural Egyptian setting Vol 5, No 4, October ISSN 1749 – 3676

EL-Adl, M; Burke, J & Little K (2009) *First-episode psychosis: primary care experience and implications for service development* Psychiatric Bulletin

Kaplan, BJ & Sadock, VA (2007) Brain Stimulation in synopsis of Psychiatry, 10th edition, ippincott Williams & Wilkins, pp:1118 - 1125

Ephesus- Wikipedia, the free encyclopedia, accessed on 03.08.11

Khaleej Times Home - ubai News, UAE News, Gulf, News, Abu Dhabi, accessed on 25.0611, 2009 v. 33, p. 165-168. [Abstract] [Full Text] [PDF]

Koyman I, Kimberlei D, Harvey S & Walsh E (2007), Br J Psychiatry, 191, s29 –39, doi 10 1192/ bjp 191.50.s29

Lopez- Junoz F, Alamao C, Cuneca C, shenn, Clervoy P, Rubio G (2005) History of discovery & clinical introduction of Chloroproimazine. Annals of Clinical Psychiatry,17 (3) 113-35

Ghalliongi (1983)Magic and Medical Science in Ancieny Egypt, The Physicians of Pharonic Egypt. Al AhramCentrefor Scientific Translation, Cairo.

Timmins, N (1994) Christopher Clunis Report: Schizophrenic made 'series of violent attacks', The Independent.

Okasha A (1993) Psychiatry in Egypt. Psychiatric Bulletin 17 :548-551.

Psychiatry in   Liverpool, 18th century PSYCHIATRY ...Journal of the Liverpool Psychiatric
     Club

Sartorius N (2004) The world Psychiatric Association global programme against stigma and
     discrimination because of schizophrenia, in Every family in the Land "revised
     edition & reprinted 2005", edited by Arthur

Sacett D (1997) Evidence based medicine. Seminars of perinatology, vol -1, issue 1, February
     1997, page 3 – 5

Yeo, M, Berzins S & Addington, D (2007) Development of an early psychosis public
     education program using the PRECEDE–PROCEED model. In Advance Access
     publication 27 October 2006Vol.22 no.5 2007, Pages 639–647 accessed on 25.06.2011.

Yung, A & McGORRY , P (2007) *Prediction of psychosis: setting the stage.* The British Journal of
     Psychiatry 2007 v. 191, p. s1-s8. [Abstract] [Full Text] [PDF]

Porter, Roy (2006). *Madmen: A Social History of Madhouses, Mad-Doctors & Lunatics.* Tempus:
     p. 14

Wikipedia. History of asylums, accessed on 6.7.2011

6

Bibliotherapy for Chinese Patients with Depression in Rehabilitation

Yang Wang

Department of Psychiatry, School of Medicine Shandong University
Psychiatric Department, Shandong Mental Health Center
China

1. Introduction

This work was aimed to explore the efficacy of bibliotherapy to the coping method and social support of patients with depression in rehabilitation, to explore influencing factors on efficacy of bibliotherapy for patients with depression in rehabilitation. A total of 362 patients with depression were randomly assigned to study group with bibliotherapy (n=184) and control group without bibliotherapy (n=178) for 4 weeks. Our results as following, at the end of study, the differences of decreased scores were significant in the two groups on retardarce factors, hopeless factors and total score of HAMD. There were significant differences on some factor scores of CMI and SSRS between after and before study in study group. In study group, there were 138 patients in efficacy group and 46 patients in inefficacy group. Stepwise regression analysis showed that the main factors that influenced the efficacy of bibliotherapy were high compliance, low age, good family economic status, high education, high using-support degree factor scores in SSRS, high recourse factor scores in CMI, without somatic disorders. In conclusion, the bibliotherapy is an effective adjutant method of rehabilitation which could improve social functions of patients with depression. The efficacy of bibliotherapy is associated with bio-psycho-social factors.

Bibliotherapy is therapy in which patients read under the guidance of professionals to cure diseases such as morbus internus and mental disorders [1]. As a novel interventional therapy for patients with depression during the rehabilitation period, the efficacy of bibliotherapy has been confirmed [2-5]. In this study, we modified the style, content, and implementation mode of traditional bibliotherapy to match Chinese depressive patients and investigated the efficacy of bibliotherapy as well as the factors that influence depressive symptoms, coping style, and social support.

2. Subjects and methods

2.1 Subjects

Subjects included patients admitted to our hospital between January, 2005, and January, 2008, who were diagnosed as having psychlepsy of mood disorder in accordance with the following inclusion criteria: (1) International Statistical Classification of Diseases and Related Health Problems (ICD-10) distributed by World Health Organization; (2) 18-35 points on the 24-item Hamilton Depression Scale (HAMD) [2], namely, these patients were in the state of slight to moderate depression; (3) attending junior middle school or over; (4) gave informed consent to subjects and their family members, or legal guardians or agents.

The exclusion criteria included the following: (1) alcohol and substance abuse or dependence; (2) obvious risks of impulsivity, self-inflicted wounds, and suicide; (3) undergoing MECT (modified electroconvulsive therapy) 6 months before inclusion; (4) myocardial infarction, angina, heart failure, severe hepatocirrhosis, renal failure, severe diabetes, aplastic anemia, angle-closure glaucoma, severe somatic diseases, organic diseases, and other diseases that may influence assessments in the trials; (5) a history of epilepsy and eclampsia; (6) participating in clinical trials for other drugs within the last month; (7) metabolic and/or other factors that may influence reading.

Discontinuation criteria included the following: (1) lack of efficacy; (2) withdrawal of informed consent; (3) noncompliance; (4) lost to follow up; (5) other harmful events that may influence the outcomes.

		Study group (n=184)	Control group (n=178)	T or X²	P
Age (years)		36.22±10.7	37.45±9.61	-0.42	0.676
Sex	Male	62(33.70)	59(33.15)	0.01	0.912
	Female	122(66.30)	119(66.85)		
Age of diagnosis (years)		28.74±6.92	27.86±8.60	0.38	0.708
Length of illness (years)		7.48±6.05	9.59±8.02	-1.00	0.323
Times of hospitalization		3.83±2.04	4.18±2.20	-0.56	0.576
HAMD total scores		±	±		
Completed rate	Completed	184(91.09)	178(88.56)	0.71	0.401
	Uncompleted	18(9.91)	23(11.44)		
Reasons for discontinuation	Lack of efficacy	5(27.78)	6(26.09)	—	0.990
	Withdrawal of consent	4(22.22)	5(21.74)		
	Lost to follow-up	4(22.22)	4(17.39)		
	Noncompliance	2(11.11)	3(13.04)		
	Other	3(16.67)	5(21.74)		

Notes: (1) the numbers in the parenthesis are the constituent ratios (%); (2) " – ", χ² value indicates Fisher precise probability χ²-test.

Table 1. Demographic and clinical features as well as trial completion rate.

In total, 403 patients were included and randomized into trial and control groups. The trial group included 202 patients, with 18 cases discontinued, leaving 184 completed cases (91.09%) aged of 22-51 years old. The age of preliminary diagnosis for these patients was 20-44 years, the length of illness was 1-25 years, and patients were admitted 1-7 times. The control group included 201 patients, with 23 cases discontinued leaving 178 completed cases (88.56%) aged 20-55 years. The age of preliminary diagnosis was 17-45 years, the length of illness was 1-26 years, and patients were admitted 1-8 times. Table 1 showed the detailed information for age, sex, age of diagnosis, length of illness, numbers of hospitalizations, demographic characteristics, such as HAMD scores, CMI scores, and SSRI scores, clinical features, and completion rates of trials.

3. Reading location

The reading room of our Mental Sanitary Center is well-suited for this study. The facility can accommodate 80 individuals and is equipped with internal facilities, many types of books, and multimedia facilities, such as cable television, a video recorder, and a VCD player.

4. Styles of bibliotherapy

Bibliotherapy utilized books, multimedia assisted lectures and television programs, and communications and symposia. Books consisted of (1) specialized books and popular science readings related to medical science, psychology, and mental science, such as Common Psychological Issues Management, Control of Unhealthy Emotion, Smoking Harm, Dietary & Health, and magazine of Mental Medicine, (2) readings related to current events and politics, such as Guangming Daily, Health Paper, Qilu Evening Paper, and World Perspectives, (3) scientific recreational readings related to science progress, interpersonal relationships, and human affections, such as Reader Digest, Family Health, and Out of Eight Hours, (4) relaxed readings related to mood adjustment and relaxation, such as celebrities biographies, interesting matters in life, short tales, novella, and cartoon and jokes.

Multimedia assisted lectures and television programs included video tapes, lectures, and internet images in which the contents consisted of hospital summaries, characteristic department introductions, common somatic diseases introduction, and pathogenesis, onset states, clinical symptoms, classification, disease course, and prognosis and treatment strategies of psychological and mental diseases. In addition, multimedia assisted lectures and television programs included television programs related to popular science, such as Lectures Room, Probe and Discovery, and Household Doctor in which the contents contained some professional knowledge of medical science related to somatic diseases, psychological problems, and mental disorders and also extended to life philosophy and manners of conducting oneself.

Communications and symposia were organized and convened regularly by professionals after the patients underwent a period of bibliotherapy. Through informal discussions and opinion exchanges, the patients shared relevant knowledge, senses, and viewpoints aroused by readings to dissolve misunderstandings.

5. Implementation mode

During the period of trials, drug treatment was conducted by clinicians and was not influenced by the trials. The subjects were randomized into groups with 9 to 12 individuals in each group. Members of each group underwent bibliotherapy every day. The length of time reading each day was 2 (or 1) hours and consisted of a free-reading period for 40 minutes and a communication period (one group is one unit) for 20 minutes. Those who learned from the readings well and had profound and real senses after reading acquired certain appraisals and rewards. Groups exchanged styles of bibliotherapy, such as books, lectures, TV programs, and symposia. The total period of bibliotherapy lasted for 30 days.

Missionaries were responsible for keeping order and controlling the trial process. In addition, missionaries provided certain assistances to the patients. For example, when professional issues could not be solved through communication among the patients, missionaries could explain and guide in an appropriate way. Also, when there was no relevant materials to meet the needs of reading, missionaries could provide materials through internet searches.

The control group patients underwent simple healing therapy that did not restrict or control the books, style, time, place, and mode of readings. The total period of control therapy lasted for 30 days.

6. Research tools

The general information scale was used, which consisted of items such as sex, age, length of illness, level of education, family history of depression, number of depression onset occurrences, number of hospitalizations, family financial status, complications from psychotic symptoms, suicide history, complications from chronic somatic diseases, type of depression onset, and therapeutic compliance. In addition, we used the HAMD [6], compiled by Hamilton, which consisted of 24 items. A total HAMD score over 17 points indicated depressive symptoms with high reliability and validity. HAMD scores decreasing by > 75% indicated healing, scores decreasing by ≥ 50% and < 75% indicated remarkable advance, scores decreasing by ≥ 25% and < 50% indicated advance, scores decreasing by > 25% (containing healing, remarkable advance, and advance) indicated effectiveness, and scores decreasing by < 25% indicated ineffectiveness. The Coping Methods Inventory (CMI) [7] was used to assess the individual coping styles, which consisted of 66 items and 6 factors (problems-solving, self-reproach, recourse, delusion, wincing, and rationalization). We also used the Social Support Rating Scale (SSRS), compiled by Xiao [8], which consisted of 10 items and 3 factors (subjective support, objective support, and availability of support) and had the high reliability and validity.

7. Research methods

At baseline, the included patients were evaluated using the general information scale, HAMD, CMI, and SSRS. After bibliotherapy, they were evaluated again using HAMD, CMI, and SSRS. Decreasing HAMD scores were indicators for the efficacy assessment, based on which the patients were divided into effective and ineffective groups. The data underwent single factor analysis among groups and subsequent multivariate progressive repression analysis.

8. Statistics

Statistical analyses, such as t-test, chi-squared test, and multivariate progressive regression analyses, were conducted using the software Statistical Analysis System (SAS) 13.0.

9. Results

9.1 HAMD scores

To investigate the amelioration of depression, the baseline factor scores or HAMD total scores and scores after intervention in the trial and control groups were compared both within and between groups, as shown in Table 2. The results showed that the factor scores

Factors	Groups	Case No.	Baseline	After intervention	T value	P value
Somatization of anxiety disorder	Trial	184	3.57±1.53	1.26±0.96	7.13	0.000
	Control	178	3.86±1.67	2.05±1.40	6.40	0.000
	T value		-0.63	-2.20		
	P value		0.535	0.033		
Body weight	Trial	184	1.48±1.47	0.87±1.01	2.95	0.007
	Control	178	1.55±1.34	0.86±0.83	3.58	0.002
	T value		-0.16	0.02		
	P value		0.874	0.983		
Cognitive disorder	Trial	184	4.74±1.94	1.91±1.65	6.38	0.000
	Control	178	4.86±1.75	2.95±1.76	6.86	0.000
	T value		-0.23	-2.05		
	P value		0.822	0.046		
Diurnal change	Trial	184	1.74±1.01	0.57±0.59	5.72	0.000
	Control	178	1.86±1.39	0.59±0.80	6.06	0.000
	T value		-0.35	-0.12		
	P value		0.732	0.902		
Retardation	Trial	184	3.17±1.78	1.39±1.23	6.51	0.000
	Control	178	3.14±1.75	2.18±1.22	4.28	0.002
	T value		0.071	-2.16		
	P value		0.943	0.036		
Sleep disorder	Trial	184	1.57±1.12	0.57±0.73	4.59	0.000
	Control	178	1.73±0.99	1.09±0.75	3.52	0.000
	T value		-0.51	-2.39		
	P value		0.610	0.022		
Sense of desperation	Trial	184	4.61±1.53	1.65±1.07	9.71	0.000
	Control	178	4.73±1.45	3.45±1.26	4.97	0.000
	T value		-0.27	-5.17		
	P value		0.791	0.000		
Total scores	Trial	184	20.87±6.07	8.22±3.25	11.33	0.000
	Control	178	21.73±5.18	13.18±3.94	11.23	0.000
	T value		-0.51	-4.63		
	P value		0.614	0.000		

Table 2. HAMD scores in trial and control groups at baseline and after bibliotherapy (mean ± SD).

and HAMD total scores of anxiety somatization, body weight, cognitive disorder, diurnal change, retardation, sleep disorder, and sense of desperation in both the trial and control groups decreased significantly (P < 0.05 for all) after intervention compared with baseline. After intervention, factor scores and HAMD total scores of anxiety somatization, cognitive disorder, retardation, sleep disorder, and sense of desperation in the trial group were significantly lower than those in control group (P < 0.05 for all). These results indicate that the depressive symptoms of patients in both the trial and control groups were remarkably ameliorated after the corresponding bibliotherapy, although the patients in trial group improved significantly more.

9.2 Decreasing HAMD scores

Decreasing HAMD scores are equal to baseline scores minus scores after intervention. To further investigate the amelioration of depression, we compared decreasing factor scores or HAMD total scores between the trial and control groups, as shown in Table 3. The results showed that decreasing HAMD scores of retardation, sense of desperation, and total scores in trial groups were significantly higher than those in control group (P < 0.05 for all), indicating that the amelioration of depression in trial groups was superior to that in control groups.

Factors	Groups	Case No.	Mean ± SD	T value	P value
Somatization of anxiety disorder	Trial	184	2.30±1.55	1.13	0.266
	Control	178	1.82±1.33		
Body weight	Trial	184	0.61±0.99	-0.26	0.796
	Control	178	0.68±0.89		
Cognitive disorder	Trial	184	2.83±2.13	1.74	0.090
	Control	178	1.91±1.31		
Diurnal change	Trial	184	1.17±0.98	-0.337	0.738
	Control	178	1.27±0.99		
Retardation	Trial	184	1.78±1.31	2.33	0.024
	Control	178	0.95±1.05		
Sleep disorder	Trial	184	1.00±1.04	1.28	0.208
	Control	178	0.64±0.85		
Sense of desperation	Trial	184	2.96±1.46	4.21	0.000
	Control	178	1.27±1.20		
Total scores	Trial	184	12.65±5.36	3.01	0.004
	Control	178	8.55±3.57		

Table 3. Decreasing HAMD scores in trial and control groups at baseline and after bibliotherapy (mean ± SD).

10. CMI scores

To investigate the improvement of coping styles, CMI factor scores in both the trial and control groups were compared between before (baseline) and after intervention, as shown in

Table 4. The results showed that factor scores of problem-solving, self-reproach, and recourse in the trial group improved significantly (P < 0.05 for all) after intervention, while those scores in the control group showed no significant differences (P > 0.05 for all) between before and after intervention. These findings indicate that the improvement of coping styles in the trial group was superior to that in the control group.

Factors	Groups	Case No.	Baseline	After intervention	T value	P value
Problem-solving	Trial	184	0.52±0.51	0.87±0.55	-2.58	0.017
	Control	178	0.50±0.51	0.64±0.58	-1.82	0.083
	T value		0.14	1.39		
	P value		0.887	0.173		
Self-reproach	Trial	184	0.78±0.60	0.48±0.59	2.61	0.016
	Control	178	0.82±0.80	0.73±0.77	1.00	0.329
	T value		-0.17	-1.22		
	P value		0.866	0.229		
Recourse	Trial	184	0.48±0.59	0.78±0.60	-3.10	0.005
	Control	178	0.50±0.67	0.55±0.67	-0.30	0.771
	T value		-0.12	1.25		
	P value		0.909	0.218		
Delusion	Trial	184	0.57±0.66	0.48±0.59	1.45	0.162
	Control	178	0.59±0.73	0.50±0.60	1.45	0.162
	T value		-0.12	-0.12		
	P value		0.902	0.903		
Wincing	Trial	184	0.65±0.71	0.57±0.66	1.45	0.162
	Control	178	0.64±0.79	0.55±0.74	1.00	0.329
	T value		0.07	0.10		
	P value		0.944	0.925		
Rationalization	Trial	184	0.13±0.34	0.17±0.39	-1.00	0.328
	Control	178	0.18±0.50	0.23±0.43	-0.44	0.665
	T value		-0.40	-0.44		
	P value		0.689	0.663		

Table 4. CMI scores in trial and control groups at baseline and after bibliotherapy (mean ± SD).

11. SSRI scores

To investigate the improvement of social support, SSRI factor scores for both the trial and control groups were compared between before (baseline) and after intervention, as shown in Table 5. The results showed that factor scores of objective support, subjective support, and availability of support in the trial group improved significantly (P < 0.05 for all) after intervention, while those scores in the control group showed no significant differences (P > 0.05 for all) between before and after intervention. These findings indicate that the improvement of social support in the trial group was superior to that in the control group.

Factors	Groups	Case No.	Baseline	After intervention	T value	P value
Objective support	Trial	184	8.13±1.91	10.09±1.81	-4.38	0.000
	Control	178	8.27±2.00	8.41±2.04	-1.82	0.083
	T value		-0.24	2.93		
	P value		0.809	0.005		
Subjective support	Trial	184	18.04±3.52	24.30±3.52	-9.24	0.000
	Control	178	18.41±3.66	19.59±3.54	-1.84	0.080
	T value		-0.34	4.48		
	P value		0.734	0.000		
Availability of support	Trial	184	7.04±1.67	10.04±1.85	-7.74	0.000
	Control	178	6.91±1.90	7.32±1.96	-1.90	0.071
	T value		0.25	4.80		
	P value		0.802	0.000		

Table 5. SSRI scores in trial and control groups at baseline and after bibliotherapy (mean ± SD)

12. Efficacy of bibliotherapy

The results showed that among 184 patients with depression during the rehabilitation period, 138 (75%) cases were effectively and 46 (25%) cases were ineffectively treated by bibliotherapy.

13. Single factor analysis of bibliotherapy efficacy

To analyze the factors that influence the efficacy of bibliotherapy in patients with depression during the rehabilitation stage, various pieces of data collected at baseline were compared between groups effectively and ineffectively treated. These data included sex, age, age at diagnosis, length of illness, degree of culture, family history of depression, number of depression onset occurrences, number of hospitalizations, family financial status, complications from psychotic symptoms, history of suicide, complications from chronic somatic diseases, type of disease onset, and therapeutic compliance. In addition, we compared CMI factor scores for problem-solving, self-reproach, recourse, delusion, wincing, and rationalization. SSRS factor scores of subjective support, objective support, and availability of support were also compared, as shown in Table 6. The results revealed significant differences (P < 0.05 for all) between effectively and ineffectively treated groups with respect to sex, age, degree of culture, family history of depression, number of depression onset occurrences, family financial status, complications from chronic somatic diseases, type of disease onset, therapeutic compliance, CMI factor scores for problem-solving, self-reproach, and recourse. We also found significant differences between effectively and ineffectively treated groups with respect to SSRS factor scores of subjective support, objective support, and availability of support.

Factors	Items	Effective group (n = 138)	Ineffective group (n = 46)	X² or T value	P value
Sex	Male	26(18.84)	35(76.09)	X²=51.02	0.000
	Female	112(81.16)	11(23.91)		
Age		31.32±9.51	38.09±8.80	T=2.48	0.017
Age of diagnosis		27.65±6.77	28.45±6.34	T=-0.41	0.684
Length of illness		6.96±4.63	8.14±5.44	T=-0.79	0.437
Degree of cultures	Junior and senior middle schools	43(31.16)	27(58.70)	X²=11.10	0.001
	Higher school or over	95(68.84)	19(41.30)		
Family history of depression	Positive	37(26.81)	27(58.70)	X²=15.46	0.000
	Negative	101(73.19)	19(41.30)		
Times of depression onset		4.52±2.19	6.14±1.78	T=-2.71	0.010
Times of hospitalization		4.30±2.29	3.68±1.89	T=0.99	0.326
Family financial status	Better	89(64.49)	13(28.26)	X²=18.33	0.000
	Worse	49(35.51)	33(71.74)		
Complications of psychotic symptom	Yes	46(33.33)	20(43.48)	X²=1.54	0.214
	No	92(66.67)	26(56.52)		
Suicide history	Yes	54(39.13)	17(36.96)	X²=0.07	0.793
	No	84(60.87)	29(63.04)		
Complications of chronic somatic disease	Yes	16(11.59)	22(47.83)	X²=27.64	0.000
	No	122(88.41)	24(52.17)		
Type of disease onset	Acute	39(28.26)	31(67.39)	X²=22.41	0.000
	Chronic	99(71.74)	15(32.61)		
Therapeutic compliance	Good	127(92.03)	25(54.35)	X²=34.10	0.000
	Bad	11(7.97)	21(45.65)		

Factors	Items	Effective group (n = 138)	Ineffective group (n = 46)	X^2 or T value	P value
CMI	Problem-solving	0.60±0.49	0.22±0.42	T=4.76	0.000
	Self-reproach	0.92±0.68	0.54±0.69	T=3.23	0.001
	Recourse	0.57±0.65	0.22±0.42	T=3.47	0.001
	Delusion	0.58±0.68	0.54±0.69	T=0.31	0.756
	Wincing	0.64±0.72	0.63±0.77	T=0.06	0.954
	Rationalization	0.14±0.39	0.17±0.49	T=-0.41	0.684
SSRS	Subjective support	8.17±1.92	7.41±2.21	T=2.22	0.028
	Objective support	18.20±3.52	16.79±3.75	T=2.30	0.023
	Availability of support	6.98±1.72	6.15±2.01	T=2.70	0.008

Note: the percentage is placed in the parenthesis.

Table 6. Single factor analysis on efficacy of bibliotherapy in the patients with depression during the rehabilitation stage

14. Multiple factor analysis of bibliotherapy efficacy

To analyze the role of bibliotherapy in factors that influence the efficacy of treatment of patients with depression in the rehabilitation stage, we conducted multivariate progressive regression analysis in which decreasing HAMD scores were dependent variables and the factors described above were independent variables. Data were evaluated according to the statistics shown in Table 7. Regression analysis revealed a total of 7 factors included in the regression formula at the significant level $\alpha = 0.05$, with the factor order based on absolute values of standard regression coefficients (namely, degree of contribution). The factor order was compliance > age > family financial status > degree of culture > SSRS factor scores of availability of support > CMI factor scores of recourse > complications from chronic somatic diseases. We obtained an R^2 value of 0.713 for the formula, which indicated that the goodness of fit by the 7 factors included into the regression formula could account for 71.3% of dependent variable variances.

15. Discussion

The therapeutic effect of bibliotherapy has long been explored by researchers. The general opinion [9] is that the choice of books reflects a channel to self-seeking of the patients and all the relvealed information such as the personality characteristics, conflict in the

Influencing factors	Repression coefficient	Standard error	Normalized regression coefficient	T value	P value
Therapeutic compliance	-0.22	0.04	-0.38	-5.41	0.000
Age	-0.20	0.04	-0.36	-4.95	0.000
Family financial status	-1.05	0.35	-0.44	-3.02	0.003
Degree of culture	2.09	0.77	0.20	2.72	0.007
Scores of availability of support in SSRS	1.88	0.74	0.18	2.52	0.013
CMI factor Scores of recourse	0.21	0.10	0.14	2.02	0.045
Complication of chronic somatic disease	0.71	0.35	0.30	2.02	0.045
constant term	10.77	2.35			

($R^2=0.713$, F=23.55, P=0.000 in the regression formula)

Table 7. Multivariate progressive regression analyses on the role of bibliotherapy in factors that influence treatment efficacy of patients with depression during the rehabilitation period.

subconsciousness, and other psychological information unknown to medical care personnel can help the evidence-based diagnosis. Clinical research issues focus on the relevant psychological problems that exist in mental patients and in during childhood growth and development. Floyd [10] studied the role of bibliotherapy in the treatment of depression in old age through two individual cases (depression caused by sadness, loneliness, and sense of guilt after spouse bereft). Felder [11] studied the efficacy of bibliotherapy in the intervention of 24 children (2-10 years of age) and their mothers with perioperative angst due to children undergoing tonsillectomy and hyperplasia adenoidectomy. Kierfeld, et al. [12] used bibliotherapy to intervene in pediatric patients with attention deficit hyperactivity disorder and oppositional defiant disorder. They found that bibliotherapy not only ameliorated the externalizing acts of the pediatric patients greatly but also improved the educational techniques and degrees of satisfaction from the children's parents, indicating that bibliotherapy had clear efficacy in the intervention of externalizing problems of pediatric patients. Buwalda, et al. [13] revealed that bibliotherapy ameliorated the symptoms and physical distress of hypochondriacs effectively. Hodgins, et al. [14] revealed that bibliotherapy prevented the recurrence of pathological gambling effectively but did not show clear improvement in the prognosis. Billich, et al. [15] revealed that bibliotherapy treatment for one month ameliorated the depressive symptoms of patients more significantly than the control group. Hahlweq, et al. [16] applied bibliotherapy to the parents of preschoolers and improved their long-term educational ability. Floyd, et al. [17] applied bibliotherapy to patients with depression in old age and conducted follow-up for 2 years. The results showed that both scores of Hamilton Rating Scale for Depression (HRSD) and

Geriatric Depression Scale (GDS) did not change upon follow-up, indicating that bibliotherapy reduced the recurrence of depression.

Coping is the cognitive and behavioral effort individuals use to manage stressful situations; it is behavior regulation corresponding to environmental variation. The main function of coping is to regulate stressful events, such as by changing the assessment of stressful events and regulating event-relevant somatic or emotional responses [18]. Some studies [19-21] indicated that coping styles regulated depression onset remarkably, and the poor coping styles were closely related to depressive mood. This current study showed clear improvement in aspects of problem solving, self-reproach, and recourse in the patients with depression during the rehabilitation period after undergoing bibliotherapy. The possible reasons for the improvement are two-fold. First, the patients acquired much professional knowledge and relevant information through contact with numerous books, TV programs, and lectures. Through these media the patients learned more ways to solve problems, learned how to manage and face negative stressors, such as adverse life events, and did not self-reproach and complain about oneself but analyzed and viewed problems in a relatively objective and comprehensive manner. Second, the patients revealed their own feelings of diseases and the misunderstanding on mental disorder to others as much as possible through communication with the wardmates and professionals, which facilitated the catharsis of inward negative mood and helped the patients learn how to ask for aids and get along with others normally. Therefore, bibliotherapy played an important role in preventing the recurrence of depression and restoring the social function of the patients, which is consistent with the results of other relevant studies [22].

Some studies [23, 24] indicated that the factor of social support was highly negatively correlated with depression. The current study showed that bibliotherapy improved the status of social support in the patients with depression during the rehabilitation period. Two possible reasons may explain the improved social supports. First, the patients with depression were characterized by wincing, loneliness, anhedonia, poor interpersonal communication, feeling of poor social support, and apparent senses of helplessness, desperation, worthlessness, and incompetence. The combination of drug therapy and intervention of bibliotherapy treated the patients with depression by pairing a pharmacological approach with helping them to acquire knowledge through reading books and watching series of videos and TV programs related to life philosophy and living experience. The bibliotherapy component relieved the anxiety disorder due to misunderstandings of mental diseases and helped the patients obtain support, restore confidence in the future, recognize their own diseases correctly, and eliminate discrimination of their own diseases. Second, during intervention, the patients had more time to communicate with wardmates and professionals on an equal platform, which helped to improve the patients' self-confidence, reacquire the sense of safety, obtain the support and aid from others, and enhance confidence and ability to study and communicate with the outside world, thus improving the status of social support.

This study followed the strong points of traditional bibliotherapy but made four specific modifications to match Chinese patients with depression during the rehabilitation period including. One modification was that in addition to professional books and popular science readings, we provided materials related to medical common sense and introduction materials related to common somatic diseases, psychological problems, and mental disorder with respect to pathogenesis, status of onset, clinical manifestation, classification, length of illness, prognosis, and treatment strategies, which could eliminate the misunderstanding of patients with mental diseases and realized their right to be informed. A second modification was that in addition to books, the contents for use in intervention were supplemented by videos, VCD, and popular science TV programs, which helped the patients to obtain the desired knowledge via visual and auditory modalities. Third, during intervention, frequency and duration of symposia and communication sessions were increased substantially, which increased the opportunity of the patients to solve their own psychological problems via communication and helped the patients practice their communication and contact abilities. Fourth, missionaries were not simply organizers and spectators but also helped the patients, such as through assisted reading, explanation and guidance of professional knowledge, and search and provision of extensive materials. This modification helped the patients to acquire knowledge and also represented the humanized management.

Single factor analysis in this study showed that good efficacy of bibliotherapy was positively correlated with individual factors, such as female, younger age, high degree of education, negative family history of depression, fewer occurrences of depression, better conditions of income, no complications from severe somatic diseases, chronic onset, high therapeutic compliance, high CMI factor scores for problem-solving, self-reproach, and recourse, as well as high SSRS factor scores for subjective support, objective support, and availability of support. However, the efficacy of bibliotherapy showed no correlation with single factors, such as length of illness, age of diagnosis, number of hospitalizations, complications from psychotic symptoms, history of suicide, CMI factor scores of delusions, wincing, and rationalization. Single factor analysis can only indicate the relationship between a single factor and efficacy of bibliotherapy in the intervention of depression, while multivariate progressive regression analysis can differentiate the main factors that have strong independent impact. In this study, the results of multivariate regression showed the following order of factors that improved the efficacy of bibliotherapy in the intervention of patients with depression during rehabilitation period: good compliance > younger age > good condition of income > high degree of cultures > high SSRS factor scores for availability of support > high CMI factor scores for recourse > no complications from severe somatic diseases. This finding was consistent with other relevant reports [25].

High therapeutic compliance was the most important factor in the efficacy of bibliotherapy. The patients with good compliance had the will to follow the intervention, studied well, and thought of and raised questions in a conscious and active manner to solve problems that they met. In these patients, unhealthy cognition was effectively treated; therefore, prognosis was improved and the risk of recurrence was reduced. This finding was consistent with other relevant reports [26, 27]. Age was the next important factor. Being influenced by degree of cultures, social and life experiences, Chinese middle-aged depressive patients did not tend to accept new things, especially those that might change their long-formed habits of mind. In contrast, younger patients had received new-style education for many years, were accustomed to contact with the external world, tended to absorb new knowledge to change and improve themselves, and tended to accept the bibliotherapy intervention, thus improving the efficacy of bibliotherapy.

This study showed that income directly influenced the efficacy of bibliotherapy in depression. The gap between the rich and the poor was large because economic development and income allocation are imbalanced in China today. In addition, the depressive patients lost some social function due to morbid or abnormal states, such as decreased volitional activity; therefore, depressive patients tended to have very low incomes. Furthermore, increasing medical-related costs have become the major economic expenditures for some families, and depression as a chronic severe mental disorder requires high medical cost. This increased cost becomes a heavy burden for some families, thus influencing the clinical symptoms and rehabilitation process of Chinese depressive patients to some extent. Therefore, in this study depressive patients may have paid more attention to economy-related issues and neglected their own depressive symptoms, coping styles, and social support, which reduced the efficacy of bibliotherapy in the intervention of depression. Degree of cultures also directly influenced the efficacy of bibliotherapy. The patients with high education backgrounds did not restrict themselves to certain reading materials but chose intended readings freely based on their preferences, tended to comprehend the implication in readings, and tended to think and summarize, which optimized bibliotherapy. Some studies [28, 29] indicated that social support and coping styles were also important factors that influenced depression. This study showed that depressive patients achieved good efficacy with bibliotherapy when they tended to use the coping style of recourse and make the best use of social support. These sorts of patients tended to take reading objectives as a style of recourse and support and combined the obtained information with their own state to correct unhealthy cognition in themselves, which improved the efficacy in the intervention of depression in an aided manner. This study also showed that the depressive patients without chronic somatic diseases were more effectively treated with bibliotherapy, likely because chronic somatic diseases as sustained stressors interact with the depressive symptoms [30]. Bibliotherapy was an aided measure of rehabilitation acting merely to improve the cognitive status of the patient with depression but could not relieve or eliminate the sustained somatic diseases; therefore, the depressive symptoms due to the worsened bodily state could not be eliminated. As readings progressed, the patients with chronic somatic diseases paid most attention to materials related to their own somatic diseases. However, the patients themselves lacked the necessary medical knowledge, so they tended to generate misunderstanding and hopelessness and form the depressive negative mood, which reduced the efficacy of bibliotherapy in the intervention of depression.

In general, this study indicated that bibliotherapy effectively improved depressive symptoms, coping styles, and social support of Chinese patients with depression during the rehabilitation period. The efficacy of bibliotherapy in the treatment of depression was influenced by many physiological, psychological, and societal factors. The contributing factors to improved efficacy of intervention included high therapeutic compliance, younger age, better family financial status, high degree of cultures, high availability of social support, use of positive coping styles such as recourse, and no chronic somatic diseases.

16. Acknowledgements

This study was supported by all nurses in department of rehabilitation on Shandong Mental Health Center, all doctors and nurses in departments of psychiatry on Shandong Mental Health Center, personnel in department of Medicine and Education on Shandong Mental Health Center, personnel in editorial board of Journal of Psychiatry and personnel in Baotuquan District of Shandong University Library.

17. Abbreviation

HAMD: Hamilton Depression Scale;
MECT: Modified electroconvulsive therapy;
CMI: Coping Methods Inventory;
SSRS: Social Support Rating Scale.

18. References

[1] Anstett RE, Poole SR. Bibliotherapy: an adjunct to care of patients with problems of living. J Fam Pract. 1983;17:845-853.

[2] Cuijpers P. Bibliotherapy in unipolar depression: a meta-analysis. J Behav Ther Exp Psychiatry. 1997;28:139-147.

[3] Smith NM, Floyd MR, Scogin F, Jamison CS. Three-year follow-up of bibliotherapy for depression. J Consult Clin Psychol. 1997;65:324-327.

[4] Fan WT, Wang Y, Xu QZ. A study of bibliotherapy in the treatment of depression. Chin J Behav Med Sci. 2006;15:336-337.

[5] Fan WT, Wang Y. A control study of bibliotherapy effects on the coping style and social supports in patients with depression in rehabilitation period. J Clin Psychosom Dis. 2007;13:213-215.

[6] Zhang MY. Psychiatric Rating Scale Manual. Changsha: Hunan Science and Technology Press; 2003. p. 121-126.

[7] Xiao JH. Response and coping style. Chin Mental Health J. 1992;6:181-183.

[8] Wang XD, Wang XL, Ma H. Mental Health Assessment Scale Manual (updated version). Beijing: Chinese Mental Health Magazine; 1999. p. 127-131.

[9] Lazarsfeld S. The use of fiction in psychotherapy. Am J Psychother. 1949;3:26-33.

[10] Floyd M. Bibliotherapy as an adjunct to psychotherapy for depression in older adults. J Clin Psychol. 2003;59:187-195.

[11] Felder PR, Maksys A, Noestlinger C. Using a children's book to prepare children and parents for elective ENT surgery: Results of a randomized clinical trial. Int J Pediatr Otorhinolaryngol. 2003;67:35-41.

[12] Kierfeld F, Dopfner M. [Bibliotherapy as a self-help program for parents of children with externalizing problem behavior]. Z Kinder Jugendpsychiatr Psychother. 2006;34:377-385; quiz 385-376.

[13] Buwalda FM, Bouman TK. Cognitive-behavioural bibliotherapy for hypochondriasis: a pilot study. Behav Cogn Psychother. 2009;37:335-340.

[14] Hodgins DC, Currie SR, el-Guebaly N, Diskin KM. Does providing extended relapse prevention bibliotherapy to problem gamblers improve outcome? J Gambl Stud. 2007;23:41-54.

[15] Bilich LL, Deane FP, Phipps AB, Barisic M, Gould G. Effectiveness of bibliotherapy self-help for depression with varying levels of telephone helpline support. Clin Psychol Psychother. 2008;15:61-74.

[16] Hahlweg K, Heinrichs N, Kuschel A, Feldmann M. Therapist-assisted, self-administered bibliotherapy to enhance parental competence: short- and long-term effects. Behav Modif. 2008;32:659-681.

[17] Floyd M, Rohen N, Shackelford JA, Hubbard KL, Parnell MB, Scogin F, Coates A. Two-year follow-up of bibliotherapy and individual cognitive therapy for depressed older adults. Behav Modif. 2006;30:281-294.

[18] Folkman S, Lazarus RS, Gruen RJ, DeLongis A. Appraisal, coping, health status, and psychological symptoms. J Pers Soc Psychol. 1986;50:571-579.

[19] Haghighatgou H, Peterson C. Coping and depressive symptoms among Iranian students. J Soc Psychol. 1995;135:175-180.

[20] Oxman TE, Hegel MT, Hull JG, Dietrich AJ. Problem-solving treatment and coping styles in primary care for minor depression. J Consult Clin Psychol. 2008;76:933-943.

[21] Kaya M, Genc M, Kaya B, Pehlivan E. [Prevalence of depressive symptoms, ways of coping, and related factors among medical school and health services higher education students]. Turk Psikiyatri Derg. 2007;18:137-146.

[22] Hodges B, Craven J, Littlefield C. Bibliotherapy for psychosocial distress in lung transplant patients and their families. Psychosomatics. 1995;36:360-368.

[23] Sorensen EA, Wang F. Social support, depression, functional status, and gender differences in older adults undergoing first-time coronary artery bypass graft surgery. Heart Lung. 2009;38:306-317.

[24] McKnight-Eily LR, Presley-Cantrell L, Elam-Evans LD, Chapman DP, Kaslow NJ, Perry GS. Prevalence and correlates of current depressive symptomatology and lifetime diagnosis of depression in Black women. Womens Health Issues. 2009;19:243-252.

[25] Fan WT, Wang Y, Meng XF. A multiple factors analysis on efficacy of bibliotherapy for patients with depression in rehabilitation. J Psychiat. 2008;21:172-175.

[26] Christensen H, Griffiths KM, Farrer L. Adherence in internet interventions for anxiety and depression. J Med Internet Res. 2009;11:e13.

[27] Sawada N, Uchida H, Suzuki T, Watanabe K, Kikuchi T, Handa T, Kashima H. Persistence and compliance to antidepressant treatment in patients with depression: a chart review. BMC Psychiatry. 2009;9:38.

[28] Crockett LJ, Iturbide MI, Torres Stone RA, McGinley M, Raffaelli M, Carlo G. Acculturative stress, social support, and coping: relations to psychological adjustment among Mexican American college students. Cultur Divers Ethnic Minor Psychol. 2007;13:347-355.

[29] Haden SC, Scarpa A. Community violence victimization and depressed mood: the moderating effects of coping and social support. J Interpers Violence. 2008;23:1213-1234.

[30] Kabir K, Sheeder J. Depression, weight gain, and low birth weight adolescent delivery: do somatic symptoms strengthen or weaken the relationship? J Pediatr Adolesc Gynecol. 2008;21:335-342.

7

Lost in the Social World: How Social Cognitive Deficits Affect Social Functioning of People with Asperger Syndrome

Mónica Figueira, Inmaculada Fuentes and Juan C. Ruiz
Faculty of Psychology, University of Valencia
Spain

1. Introduction

Were we to visualise autism spectrum disorders as a continuum, Asperger syndrome (AS) would be situated at one of its extremes. What appears to determine each individual's position in this continuum is his or her symptomatology. In the case of AS symptomatology presents itself more discretely. According to Barthélemy (2000), the abovementioned symptomatology can be grouped in three major areas: a) difficulties in development of social interaction; b) difficulties in verbal and nonverbal communication; and c) presence of fixated interests, routines or rituals and repetitive behaviours. Being a developmental disorder, symptoms vary according to age. While some features tend to disappear with time, others only appear in a posterior stage of development and the changes can be spectacular (Frith, 2006). Citing Frith (2006, p. 16), "the autism affects the development, as well as the development affects autism". Besides the variability on behaviour, there is also great diversity at a cognitive level, which can range from a medium or superior level of intelligence to profound mental retardation. Approximately 60% of autistic children present an Intelligence Quotient [IQ] under 50; 20% between 50 and 70 and 20% above 70 (Ritvo & Freeman, 1978). More recent data points to the presence of mental retardation in 75% of the cases (Barthélemy, 2000). The existence of a normal level of intelligence (IQ above 70) is the variable that distinguishes classic cases of autism from those considered as the "High Functioning Autism" or the person with AS.

However, it is not yet clear if there are significant differences between "High Functioning Autism" and AS from the point of view of cognitive and behavioural profile. According to the working group that is preparing the fifth edition of DSM-V (American Psychiatric Association [APA], 2010), the current field of research reflects two views: 1) That AS is not substantially different from other forms of 'high functioning' autism; i.e. Asperger's is the part of the autism spectrum with good formal language skills and good (at least verbal) IQ, noting that 'high functioning' autism is itself a vague term, with underspecification of the area of 'high functioning' (performance IQ, verbal IQ, adaptation or symptom severity); 2) That AS is distinct from other subgroups within the autism spectrum: e.g. Klin et al. (2005) suggest the lack of differentiating findings reflects the need for a more stringent approach, with a more nuanced view of onset patterns and early language.

Additionally, several studies have pointed to the non-existence of distinctive criteria at a cognitive and behavioural level to differentiate between these two clinical conditions (Manjiviona & Prior, 1999; Miller & Ozonoff, 2000; Ozonoff, South & Miller, 2000). Some researchers defend that what distinguishes a person with 'high functioning autism' from another with AS is the presence (High Functioning Autism) or not (AS) of a delay in the development of language in childhood. Since this criterion is not very significant in terms of cognitive and behavioural profiles (that is similar in both groups) and since there is still no consensus in scientific literature whether these two designations are referring to a unique disorder or not, in the present work we will only utilize the term AS to designate the group of people that belong to the autism spectrum disorder that have a normal or above normal IQ, independently of the delay in language development in childhood.

Now focusing on AS, we can say that one of it's characteristic features is social impairment, but social cognition, or the ability to understand the social world around us, appears to be also affected. Nonetheless, the relationship between social cognition and social functioning in AS still remains unclear. The aim of this chapter is to describe the concept of social cognition, analyse how different aspects of the concept may be affected in AS and explore how social functioning may be impaired in this clinical condition. Possible connections between these two types of impairment will also be examined.

2. Social cognition in Asperger syndrome

In general terms, social cognition is related to the way each person understands and interprets social situations, i.e. it involves the information that is perceived from the world around us, the interpretations that we make from this information and the way we react to the social world in accordance with that initial interpretation. One of the most complete and utilized definitions of social cognition is given by Brothers (1990) and refers to the mental operations underlying social interactions, which include processes involved in perceiving, interpreting and generating responses to the intentions, dispositions, and behaviours of others. According to Striano & Reid (2009), social cognition involves our ability to predict, monitor, and interpret the behaviours and mental states of other people.

Social cognition includes various domains, such as emotional processing, theory of mind (ToM), social perception, social scheme, and attributional style. Emotional processing refers broadly to aspects of perceiving and using emotion. Emotion perception has been the most extensively studied social cognitive process and refers to the ability to infer emotional information from facial expressions, vocal inflections, or the combination of both (Horan et al., 2008). Theory of mind refers to the ability to understand that others have mental states that differ from one's own and the capacity to make correct inferences about the content of those mental states. Processes typically associated with theory of mind involve the ability to understand false beliefs, hints, intentions, metaphor, and irony (Horan et al., 2008). Social perception refers to a person's ability to judge social cues from contextual information and communicative gestures, including awareness of the roles, rules, and goals that typically characterize social situations and guide social interactions. Social perception can also refer to one's perception of relationships between people, in addition to perception of cues that are generated by a single person (Fiske, 1992). Social scheme is linked to social perception and refers to the ability to identify the components that characterize a social situation. The identification of social signs requires knowledge of what is typical in a social situation. It is the social scheme that determines how to act, what is our role and the role of others in a social situation and what are the rules that should be followed and the goal of that situation (Ruiz et al., 2006). Finally, attributional style refers to how individuals characteristically explain the causes for positive and negative events in their lives (Horan et al., 2008).

In our daily routine we are constantly using social cognitive processes because we depend on them to feel socially situated, to understand social situations and others, to take perspective and to understand what others are expecting of us. All this seems extremely simple and normal. Nonetheless, things are different when social cognition is affected and AS is a disorder where this is very much so, with considerable deficits in emotional processing, social perception and theory of mind.

2.1 Emotional processing

It is important to analyse two aspects: 1) to understand how people with AS process emotions, and 2) to present studies that have been developed dealing with face processing that can explain difficulties in emotional processing in AS.

Different diagnostic criteria of AS describe, clinically substantial difficulties for comprehension, expression and regulation of emotions, e.g. lack of social and emotional reciprocity (APA, 2002); social and emotional behaviour inadequate for the social situation and limited facial expression that is inadequate for the situation (Gillberg, 1991); difficulties in perceiving feelings and emotions in others, limited facial expression and inability to read emotions through facial expressions, as well as transmitting messages through gaze. It is also common for people with AS to have a limited vocabulary to describe their emotional state, mostly when the emotions are more complex (Attwood, 2009). Most studies that have been carried out on emotional processing in AS have focused on the identification of basic emotions and the results have been contradictory, with some authors saying that there is a difficulty in recognizing basic emotions through facial expressions, voice tone or both (Celani et al., 1999; Deruelle et al., 2004; Hobson 1986a, 1986b; Kuusikko et al., 2009; Loveland et al., 1995; Macdonald et al., 1989; Yirmiya et al., 1992) while others maintain that there are no difficulties in this area (Baron-Cohen et al., 1993; Boucher et al., 2000; Grossman et al., 2000). On the other hand, studies that have evaluated the identification of more complex emotions have demonstrated a greater and more consistent evidence of the difficulty to recognize these types of emotions (Attwood, 2009; Baron-Cohen et al., 1999; Baron-Cohen et al., 2001; Capps et al., 1992; Golan et al., 2006; Golan et al., 2008; Happé, 1994; Shamay-Tsoory, 2008; Yirmiya et al., 1992).

The emotions and feelings of other's are interpreted either through voice tone, or through facial and corporal expressions (Kuusikko et al., 2009). We will focus only on facial expressions to introduce the second question, face processing. People with AS have difficulties in reading facial expressions because they process faces as they do objects and they seem to pay attention only to the individual components of a face, which affects the interpretation of emotional expression. Face processing can be described as the central source of information about the emotion and the ability to recognize the emotional state of others requires the ability to pay attention and to focus on relevant information (Kuusikko et al., 2009). Typical errors in AS are, on the one hand, not distinguishing between which keys are relevant and which are not and, on the other, wrongly interpreting those keys. Several studies using advanced technology such as eye-tracking to evaluate visual attention to faces, have reported that people with AS show reduced attention to eyes, which is the region of the face providing more information about the expression of different emotions (Baron-

Cohen et al., 1997b; Bassili, 1979; Calder et al., 2000). This has also been reported in a case study of a 15-month-old baby (Klin & Jones, 2008). Chawarska & Shic (2009) verified that AS children moved away their gaze from faces progressively with age, and they did not focus their gaze on relevant regions of faces (like the ocular region), focusing more on external characteristics. Similar conclusions were reported in several other studies (Freeth et al., 2010; Klin et al., 2002b; Pelphrey et al., 2002; Speer et al., 2007). With regard to the use of facial information to infer emotions, Spezio et al. (2007) verified that people with AS use more information from the mouth rather than the eye region to infer emotions. Other studies have reported that people with AS are less capable than people with typical development of inferring information from the eyes of another person (Baron-Cohen et al., 1997a; Baron-Cohen et al., 2001). Hence, using information transmitted by the eyes to know what another person is thinking and feeling, poses problems for people with AS. On the one hand, they do not look very much in the eyes of other people. On the other, when they are capable of establishing eye contact, the interpretation that they make about the information provided from the other person's eyes is not very efficient (Attwood, 2009). In the light of these studies about emotion identification and face processing, it is important to reflect on the possible relationship between emotional processing and face processing. Considering those studies that report deficits in face processing and postulate that people with AS tend to focus their gaze on external characteristics, not paying much attention to faces and that when they do pay it, tending to focus more on the mouth rather than the eye region and knowing that the eye region is the richest in information about emotions that are transmitted through faces, we can venture that the deficit in processing emotions can be due to inadequate face processing. To conclude, it is important to establish what implications these deficits have (whether in face processing or in emotion processing) in the life of a person with AS. If such a person cannot understand the emotions that are expressed by the people around her, she surely cannot know how to react to those people, because she is not capable of interpreting the signs around her, she does not know what to think, say or do. This being the case, it is very common for a person with AS to think, say and do awkward things that are misinterpreted by others. The person with AS knows when her speech or behaviour is inadequate, and this makes her feel socially incompetent. Being aware of her own difficulties and limitations, the person with AS feels like she does not fit in the social world, and this encourages her to avoid social interaction and leads to social isolation. She becomes closed in her own world, where she knows that no one will bother her and where she can have her desired peace, aware of the confusion inherent in the world of social relationships.

2.2 Theory of mind

As previously mentioned, ToM refers to the ability to recognize and understand what others think, wish or what their intentions are, with the goal of understanding and predicting their behaviour (Attwood, 2009). Several studies have demonstrated that both children and adults with AS present difficulties in the abilities of ToM (Baron-Cohen, 2001; Bowler, 1992; Frith, 2006; Happé, 1994; Kalland et al., 2002; Kalland et al., 2008; Leslie, 1987; Ozonoff et al., 1991; Ponnet et al., 2004; Spek et al., 2010). As Frith (2006) defends, these persons are not programmed to reflect automatically about the mental states of others and present difficulties in "putting themselves into others' shoes" or taking perspectives. For that reason, Baron-Cohen (1995) states that they are mindblind. One of the consequences of deficits in theory of mind is the tendency to make literal interpretations of everything that is said by others. Metaphors, sarcasm and irony also generate much confusion. This occurs because these people are unable to understand the existing incongruence between what is said and facial expression, voice tone and context (Kleinman et al., 2001; Rutherford et al., 2002). ToM deficits also affect problem solving, due to difficulties in thinking about the point of view and priorities of others, limited abilities in persuasion, a tendency to polarize and to be rigid and inflexible and resistance to changing opinion and decision (Attwood, 2009). Another question related to ToM which affects the daily life of a person with AS is that these people are extremely sincere, putting this above anything else, including the emotions, opinions and feelings of others. People with AS do not know when to refrain from making comments that, although true, may hurt others, and all this is due to the fact that they are not able to infer the mental states of others or "put themselves in others' shoes". There are different levels of ToM and tasks have been created to measure ToM accordingly. There are first order tasks, that consist simply of making inferences about the mental states of others, e.g. 'Where does Sally think her doll is?'; second order tasks, that consist of attributing more complex mental states to others, e.g. 'What does Sally think that Anne is thinking?', and finally advanced ToM tasks, that consist of interpreting more complex social situations, based on subtle information (Spek et al., 2010). Children with AS can pass first and second order ToM tasks, but not at the age that was expected. They only can pass them at a more advanced stage of their development (Bowler, 1992; Happé, 1993; Happé, 1995). Adults with AS also do not present difficulties in these kinds of tasks (first and second order tasks) (Baron-Cohen, 2001; Bowler, 1992; Happé, 1994; Ozonoff et al., 1991). But this does not mean that they are able to function adequately in social situations, because in our daily lives we have to face more subtle social information, which is harder to interpret (Ozonoff et al., 1991). Hence, even adults with AS that can pass first and second order tasks of ToM, present difficulties in passing more advanced tasks of ToM (Baron-Cohen et al., 1997a; Baron-Cohen et al., 1997b; Happé, 1994; Kalland et al., 2008; Spek et al., 2010).

Given the above-mentioned studies, it is possible to say that people with AS present deficits in ToM, because at any level of development there is always an inability to pass tasks of ToM in keeping with their stage of development, which means that throughout their development, they will always demonstrate incomprehension of what people around them are thinking or feeling, resulting in their not knowing what to say or how to react to such people.

2.3 Social perception

While people with typical development can notably figure out social cues that indicate the feelings and thoughts of others and can understand these, as if their minds prioritise social cues above anything else, people with AS perceive more information from the physical world than from the social world (Attwood, 2009). Moreover this occurs in very early stages of development. Klin & Jones (2008) reported a case of a 15-month-old infant that suggested that the viewing patterns of the child with autism were driven by the physical contingences of the stimuli rather than by their social context. Studies with older children (around 5 years old) verified that while neurotypical children prefer hearing the voice of their mothers (social stimuli), children with an autism spectrum disorder (ASD) prefer hearing sounds that are not related to persons (non social stimuli) (Klin, 1991; 1992). Similar conclusions were obtained by Mongillo et al. (2008) and by Sheppard et al. (2010). Attempting to explain this preference we can say that the social world appears to be too confusing and difficult to interpret for people with AS. Hence it is much easier to pay attention to non-social information because this type of information does not need to be deciphered according to some secret code that only people with typical development seem to master. On the other hand, difficulties in social perception can also be related to another question, that is the attention that is paid to social context. People with AS do not use context when processing social stimuli. Beyond having difficulties in utilizing information coming from context during information processing, people with AS invest more time on less relevant characteristics, paying more attention to details than to the big picture (Happé & Frith, 2006; Klin et al., 2002a). All this leads to a deficit in perception of socially relevant stimuli. Linked to this is the concept of central coherence, which refers to the ability to integrate information in context (Frith, 2006). Further to the deficit in ToM and in emotional processing, in AS there is also weak central coherence, i.e. when people with AS are processing information they are excellent at fixating on detail but present serious difficulties in understanding the general perspective or the context (Frith & Happé, 1994). Weak central coherence explains some difficulties felt by people with AS at a social level. Having a weak central coherence means that people cannot easily differentiate between what is relevant and what is superfluous in a social situation. For example, when a person with typical development goes into a large space, where there are a lot of people with a lot of social activity, the brain is inundated with a huge amount of new information, but is capable of identifying and selecting only that which is important and socially relevant. People with typical development have a system of priorities and the usual priority is to focus on people and on conversations and not on the drawing on the rug on the floor or on the decorative flowers or the lights that are illuminating the place. People with AS are less capable of determining what is important in social terms and what is not. Hence, they will probably pay more attention to the rug, to the flowers or to the lights because it is much easier to pay attention to physical stimuli rather than to social stimuli. After the event, people with typical development tend to remember the people, conversations and emotions felt and forget socially irrelevant information. Conversely, people with AS will not remember such detail, but instead will remember a lot of details that other people would consider unimportant (Attwood, 2009). It is possible to distinguish two important aspects of social perception. On the one hand, people with AS present difficulties in perceiving the world around them in a general way, i.e. they can not get the big picture because they prefer to focus on details. On the other hand, looking only at the information they perceive, they prefer to focus on non-social rather than socially relevant information.

All this has implications in the life of the person with AS, because by focusing on socially irrelevant rather than socially relevant information, the person with AS will present difficulties in interpreting social situations and will not know how to react to these. The behaviour of the person with AS will be socially inadequate. Being aware of their social maladjustment, people with AS avoid social contact, preferring to be isolated in their own worlds.

3. Social functioning in Asperger syndrome

3.1 Social functioning on adolescence and early adulthood

In adolescence, teenagers start to become more interested in social relationships and become concerned with being socially accepted in their peer group as well as attaching more importance to friends. This happens with most adolescents, even with those that do not have friends, but would like to, like teenagers with AS (Patrick, 2008). Nonetheless, wanting to have friends is not the same as knowing how to enter into a relationship (Sicile-Kira, 2008) and this is where we can distinguish a teenager with AS from one without. People with AS do not know how to interrelate and consider this to be extremely difficult. Attwood (2009) mentions that some adults with AS feel that social interactions seem to employ a completely different language, like a foreign language that has not been taught to them by anyone and for which they have no translation. According to Sicile-Kira (2008), things get more complicated because different rules seem to exist according to different social relationships. Given the existence of these different types of relationships, each one with its own set of rules that seems to be obvious to people with typical development but less so obvious to those with AS, the latter has to learn an infinitude of rules and social skills that are suited to different kinds of social relationships (with parents, with friends, with teachers, with neighbours) and to different kinds of social situations (in job interviews, on a date). There are a lot of social interactions that people with AS have to face throughout their lives and each one of them requires specific social skills and it is precisely here where they have difficulty in knowing which one is appropriate for each situation. Learning social skills is an extremely hard and exhausting task for such people because the process consists of multiple attempts and errors, and thousands of misunderstandings occur in interpersonal relations. As Sicile-Kira (2006) points out, AS can be considered a disability of social misunderstandings. These constant misunderstandings lead the adolescent or the adult with AS to see the social world as an ocean of impossible navigation. The unpredictability of the social world is the cause of a constant state of anxiety governing the lives of a lot of these people and that is why many prefer to auto segregate in order to avoid confusion and suffering.

3.2 Social skills

Social skills are the capabilities that we are expected to use to interact with others in our society. They are based on the social norms of our society and tell us what attitudes and behaviours are considered to be normal, acceptable and expected in a particular social situation (Patrick, 2008). Social skills are important because they allow us to interact with each other with predictability, so that we can more readily understand each other and be understood. People who have well-developed social skills are generally viewed by others in their society as competent and successful. They also tend to be well liked by others, while those who struggle to master the social skills are often viewed by society as inept.

Entering adulthood is hard for most people. Nonetheless, it is particularly difficult for a person with AS because living independently requires a lot of abilities that they seem to have difficulties in acquiring, given their special characteristics. This is a propitious moment to start honing social skills. Nonetheless, while adolescents with typical development acquire these skills easily as part of a natural development process, people with AS face far more difficulties at this stage. People with AS fail to learn adequate social skills and this can lead to isolation, feelings of loneliness, frustration, rejection, and poor self-esteem.

According to Patrick (2008), social skills consist of three elements: social intake, internal process, and social output. Social intake refers to our seeing and understanding the words, vocal inflection, body language, eye contact, posture, gestures, and other cultural behaviours that accompany a social message. Internal process refers to our interpretation of the social message in addition to recognizing and managing our own emotions and reactions. Social output refers to how we respond to the message through our own words, vocal inflection, body language, eye contact, posture, gestures, and cultural behaviours.

Attempting to explain difficulties in social skills felt by the person with AS and taking the above-mentioned elements as a point of analysis, we can say that the person with AS fails early on the first element, that is social intake.

This is related to the fact that they present deficits in social cognition. Information processing is more selective and more focused on details and not on the global context or on the big picture. Additionally, there is a preference for perceiving socially irrelevant rather than socially relevant stimuli. So, if people with AS prefer to focus their attention on physical stimuli (socially irrelevant) and not on social stimuli it is perfectly normal that they will not be paying attention to vocal inflection, body language, posture and to all non verbal communication elements that are transmitted in a social interaction. Since they are not paying attention to this type of information, they fail early on in the first stage of the process of putting social skills into practice. And if there is a failure at this first stage, then it is obvious that everything later in the process will be affected, i.e. the person that does not correctly perceive social stimuli, will not be able to process them at an internal level, so will therefore not know how to adequately react. This results in extremely deficient social skills and lack of adjustment to social situations.

It is a fact that people with AS present a deficit in social skills, but can these be learned? The biggest problem with learning social skills in AS is the fact that these people fail on the application of social rules to daily situations. And this is a very hard task because we live in an age where social norms are changing at a rapid rate and where it is virtually impossible for any human being to know and master every social skill required for every setting, since one way of acting in a specific situation may not be adequate for another one if the context is different (Patrick, 2008).

Nonetheless, a lot of adolescents and young adults with AS can improve their social skills, albeit slowly. Because changes in social behaviour are so difficult, every little gain or advance must be highly valued. Grandin, an adult with AS, asks, "Does this give us an excuse to put aside the effort it takes to function socially? No. It just means that our social learning never stops" (Grandin & Barron, 2005, p.24).

3.3 Communication

Even if a person with AS has exhibited some exceptional abilities at language since childhood, such as using a rich and complex vocabulary, that could include technical terms (usually associated with a particular interest) and some expressions that are used only by adults, these persons also present a lot of difficulties on a communicational level. One of the most visible is the incapability of modifying language in accordance with social circumstances. Pragmatics is the area that studies the use of language in social contexts and this is extremely affected in AS. Another language characteristic of people with AS is prosody, i.e. the melody of speech, in particular, voice tone, that in some persons can sound strange because it is perceived as flat and monotonous. When we hear a person with AS speaking, peculiarities of the tone, inflexion and rhythm of the voice are evident (Fine et al., 1991; Paul et al., 2005; Shriberg et al., 2001). Prosodic function involves three aspects: grammatical, pragmatic and affective. Grammar seems not to be affected in AS. Nonetheless the prosody of people with AS is strange at a pragmatic and affective level (Shriberg et al., 2001) because the speech of these persons does not transmit the degree of social and emotional information that is expected. People with AS also have difficulties in understanding the importance of voice tone, inflexions or the accentuation of certain words when they are listening to someone else talking (Koning & Magill-Evans, 2001). These subtle keys are very important if we want to identify the different intentions, thoughts and emotions of others. Another speech characteristic that seems to be affected in AS is the volume of the voice, that may be too high or too low for the situation. A too-high tone of voice is extremely irritating to family members and hard for teachers, who are constantly trying to maintain silence in the classroom (Attwood, 2009). As for the fluidity of verbal expression in AS, Attwood (2009) maintains that these people either speak too much or not at all. If the theme is of particular interest, conversation gives way to an authentic verbiage and incessant questions about the topic. In this process of authentic verbiage, it is common that people with AS do not interpret signs that are telling them to stop talking. On the other hand, there are also people with AS that appear mute for periods of time (Gillberg & Billstedt, 2000). This seems to be due to anxiety, which affects verbal fluidity. Sometimes, during a conversation with a person with AS, there are moments when it seems that there has been a malfunction in the communication transmission. The person turns quiet; thinking about what to say next and, in order to get concentrated, avoids looking at the face of the other person. Such behaviour can confound the interlocutor, who is waiting for an immediate answer and begins to wonder if they should interrupt the thoughts of the person with AS in order to re-establish the dialogue (Attwood, 2009).

Normally, people with AS do not like to be interrupted when they are talking, yet they usually interrupt others or continue talking when they should not do so (Grandin, 1995). This normally happens because they are not able to interpret the signs that indicate that they should not interrupt or continue talking. During a conversation between people with typical development, it is expected that the person listening shows signs of paying attention to what is being said and communicates this with gestures and other elements of nonverbal communication. These behaviours confirm the sensation of communication and being in tune with the speaker. These signs of nonverbal communication are less evident when one of the interlocutors is a person with AS. The signs that demonstrate agreement and the sensation of listening with attention and empathising are not present in the communication process of a person with AS (Attwood, 2009). It is also common that, during a conversation, the person with AS frequently changes the topic of conversation, unaware of the fact that the logical connection between themes is not evident to her interlocutor. These conversations, or rather monologues, seem to be unstructured and are perceived by the interlocutor as an offloading of thoughts and experiences without any coherence or relevance to the particular situation. The person with AS is unable to perceive the perspective of an interlocutor who is trying to follow the logic of the conversation while at the same time wondering about the purpose of what is being said. In conversations with people with AS, comments engaging the interlocutor, such as "what do you think about this?" or "have you ever had any similar experience?"are always missing.

Furthermore, people with AS do not follow conventional norms of initiating, maintaining and finishing a conversation. They may start an interaction with a comment that does not fit in that particular situation. For example, a child with AS may come across an unknown person at the supermarket and initiate a conversation saying "do you have a telescope?" then continue with a monologue that shows an encyclopaedic knowledge of astronomy. Once the conservation is initiated, it seems that there is no way of stopping until the child gets to the end of what seems to be a well rehearsed talk about that specific topic. The person with AS is not conscious of the effect produced by her monologue on the interlocutor and does not perceive the signs of confusion and desire to finish the conversation that are emitted by the other person. It looks as if the person with AS just talks, does not listen and is oblivious to the non verbal signs regulating the flux of communication. During the conversation, the person with AS does not appreciate the context or the social norms. Another difficulty felt by the person with AS arises when the conversation needs to be re-established. When a conversation becomes confuse, the natural reaction of people with typical development is to ask for clarification in order to keep the conversation on the topic. However, a person with AS has doubts about what to say, and does not have the courage to admit this or that she is confused. She remains silent for a long time thinking about what she should say or changes the subject for another one that is more familiar and of interest to her (Adams et al., 2002). Contrary to what happens in their monologues, when people with AS participate in a conversation that is of no interest to them or that has not been initiated by them, they become resistant and do not take part in the conversation, because they consider that they do not have anything to learn with it. Hence, they do not even waste time speaking or hearing what others have to say (Paul & Sutherland, 2003). This is why they appear to have no appreciation of chatting, which does not have a defined goal, because they do not understand its utility (Sicile-Kiran, 2008).

3.4 Communication skills
Communication skills are a set of capabilities that we use to exchange information, thoughts, attitudes, ideas and feelings clearly and accurately. It is through communication that we get the information we need to survive (Patrick, 2008). Communication is made up of the words we use, how we say the words, and our nonverbal communication. The words we use come from our language, how we say the words is determined by the paralinguistic rules of our language, and nonverbal communication is made up of the wordless messages we send through our body language (Windle & Warren, 1999). The speaker to emphasize communication, with the purpose of providing clarity for the listener, uses paralinguistic cues. Communication requires a speaker and a listener. It is the role of the speaker to send a clear and concise message. On the other hand, it is the role of the listener to receive and correctly interpret the message sent by the speaker. In order to become effective communicators, we must develop the skills required by both the speaker and the listener (Patrick, 2008). The speaker must be able to convey a clear and concise message. In order to do this the speaker must have a good command of our language, the paralinguistic cues that support our spoken language, and knowledge of nonverbal communication. She must also be concerned that her message is heard and understood by the listener. It is the responsibility of the speaker to construct the message so that the listener can understand it. This means the speaker must have the capacity to see the perspective of the listener and be able to address his point of view. On the other hand, listening is the key to receiving messages and the listener is the person responsible for receiving the message. Therefore, listening is a combination of hearing what another person says and psychological involvement with the person who is speaking (Windle & Warren, 1999). Listening requires more than hearing just words. It requires a desire to understand another human being, an attitude of respect and acceptance, and a willingness to try to see things from another person's point of view (Patrick, 2008). Listening to understand is a difficult task, which requires specific skills like giving full attention to the other person, observing the other person, and then thinking about what the other person is trying to communicate (Bolton,

1979). Giving full attention to the speaker means that the listener must pay attention to both the verbal and nonverbal message and must attempt to take the perspective of the speaker and try to see the communication from the speaker's point of view. According to Patrick (2008), it is through the language (what is conveyed by words), paralinguistic cues (how we say it), and nonverbal communication (corporal language that accompanies what is being said) that we can understand what the speaker is trying to communicate and that is why we must pay special attention to each one of these aspects.

Firstly, our language is the socially shared and agreed upon system of communication made up of symbols that we use with other people to express and exchange ideas, thoughts, attitudes, facts and feelings.

Paralinguistic cues are the features of our speech that are used to emphasize communication for the purpose of providing clarity for the listener. These features include pitch, loudness, rhythm, stress and intonation of the voice. Paralinguistic cues involve how something is said, not the content of what is said. Pitch refers to the sound of the voice, that can be high or low; loudness refers to the volume of the voice, which can be loud or soft; rhythm refers to the metric pattern of speech which differs within each language, and stress refers to the emphasis placed upon which word is stressed. Paralinguistic cues increase the clarity of the intended message; therefore they are essential for understanding and being understood by others.

Nonverbal communication is the process of communicating by sending and receiving wordless messages. These messages are sent through facial expressions, eye contact, gestures, body language, and posture.

In a study about communication of feelings and attitudes, Mehrabian (1972) discovered that verbal language, i.e. the words that we use, account for 7 percent of all meaning in communication that involves feelings and attitudes, attributing up to 93 percent of meaning to other variables. Paralinguistic cues are one of these variables and account for as much as 38 percent of meaning and nonverbal communication accounts for 55 percent of all meaning when discussing feelings and attitudes. In other words, it is the nonverbal communication that transmits the most meaning.

People communicate through nonverbal communication even when they might not want to communicate. The human body when awake will communicate even without permission. As one of Watzlawick's five axioms of communication states, „One cannot not communicate" (Watzlawick et al., 1967), because we are constantly communicating, since our body is always sending messages, verbal or nonverbal. Since it is impossible not to communicate, the question that we have to put is: „how should we communicate?". And we can choose to communicate effectively. To accomplish that, a person must be able to listen as well as to speak, but that is not the end of the story. A person can have the most highly developed language, but unless he or she is able to apply that language to social settings, the effectiveness of communication will be impeded (Patrick, 2008). This is what seems to happen in AS and that is why it is important to analyse which communication skills they have developed and which ones pose more difficulties.

The only communication skill that seems to be well developed in AS is the one that is related to verbal language or to the use of the words, not only with the purpose of transmitting messages, but also in the reception of verbal messages. This communication ability seems to be intact in AS (Tager-Flusberg et al., 2005), because, as mentioned earlier, these people have well developed language and that is why they are able to adequately transmit and receive verbal messages. This being the case, the problem lies with the other two components of communication that are supposed to accompany verbal messages (Klin & Volkmar, 1997; Paul & Landa, 2008; Tager- Flusberg et al., 2005). People with AS have difficulties in interpreting paralinguistic cues and are unable to pay attention to all nonverbal messages that are transmitted through facial expressions, gestures, and corporal posture. This explains the difficulties felt by a person with AS when assuming the role of listener. Nonetheless, when such a person assumes the role of speaker there are also difficulties, such as being unable to accompany the verbal message with paralinguistic cues and signs of nonverbal communication that can support it. Until now we have seen which communication skills people with AS have difficulty with, nonetheless it is important to offer an explanation to better understand why they have these difficulties. As far as paralinguistic cues are concerned, a person with AS pays no attention to these subtleties of the language, and consequently cannot interpret their meaning. On the other hand, when a person with AS assumes the speaker's role, she does not use paralinguistic cues, because she does not recognize their importance and is unaware that they are useful to emphasize what she is saying in words. The inability to adequately use paralinguistic cues can also be related to typical linguistic problems in AS which have been mentioned earlier, like prosody and lack of rhythm in speech (speaking always with the same voice tone), which makes it difficult to add paralinguistic cues to the speech of these persons.

With regard to nonverbal communication, people with AS present difficulties in interpreting the signs of the nonverbal communication (Sicile-Kira, 2008) that support the verbal message. Conscious of the fact that these signs have a social nature, and taking into account what has been referred to in the previous topic on social perception, we can say that people with AS do not pay attention to socially relevant information, so it is only natural that they do not take notice of facial expressions or the body language utilized by the speaker.

Considering that people with AS do not attend to either paralinguistic cues or nonverbal communication signs, and remembering the Mehrabian (1972) data, the person with AS only understands 7 percent of the meaning of the whole message, because she only interprets correctly what is said by words and does not care about paralinguistic cues and nonverbal communication elements, that together account for 93 percent of the meaning of the message being conveyed.

In the light of these values, we can say that people with AS present difficulties in communication skills, because they cannot correctly interpret a large part of the message that is transmitted in the communication process. Furthermore, these limitations also apply when they are in the role of speaker, but in a different way. If they do not interpret the signs of non-verbal communication in others, it is because they do not value them and maybe do not even notice that they are important in the communication process. Consequently, if their importance is not recognized, emitting signs of nonverbal communication will not be a concern for these people when they are transmitting a message.

To conclude, the messages of people with AS are not accompanied by either paralinguistic cues or nonverbal communication signs. Hence these messages that are transmitted will always be poor in informative terms because they will depend only on the verbal message, i.e. the person only says what she wants to say without emphasizing it either with paralinguistic cues or nonverbal communication elements, such as an adequate facial expression, gestures or a corporal posture depending on what is being said.

In summary, we can say that in the communication process, messages are always misinterpreted by people with AS, as are the messages that are transmitted by these people (poor in informative terms).

Further to the above-mentioned difficulties in communication skills, there is another aspect that is extremely affected in AS, either as the speaker or as the listener in the communication process. This is the ability to ensure that the message is correctly heard and understood by the listener, assuming the person with AS takes on the role of speaker, and the ability to show a speaker that what is being said, is being heard and understood, when the person with AS is the listener.

Both abilities are deficient in people with AS, because they require the ability to take on the perspective of the others and to see things from their point of view. Such skills are blatantly missing in people with AS and are related to the component of social cognition known as theory of mind.

3.5 Relation between communication skills and social skills

Social and communication skills are related through pragmatics. According to Marcondes (2000), pragmatics is the area of linguistics that studies language in the context of its use in communication, studying the existing relations between the signs and the speakers, describing the use that these make of the linguistic in different communication situations. Frith (2006) maintains that pragmatics includes rules for conversations and communication acts. The conversational rules include turn-taking, levels of formality, and topic maintenance. With regard to the communication act, it includes the appropriate rate of speech, pitch, stress, intonation, loudness, quantity of information, quality of information, and directness of the information.

It is pragmatics that sets the rules for the social use of linguistics and it is only when the speaker and listener both have a command of these rules that clear, effective and meaningful communication can occur. All this reverberates at a social level, because when communication is made effectively, social interactions turn out well. Nonetheless, people with AS seem to have difficulties in understanding and following these rules, and this may result in deficient communication and, consequently, affect their social interactions.

As mentioned previously regarding communication and social skills, we could say that, although these two are united by pragmatics, communication skills could be seen as an integrated and necessary element in good development of social skills, inasmuch as the latter seems to be a wide domain of skills which could include the former.

However, although social skills are a wider field than communication skills, this does not mean that communication skills are less important, because they are a necessary and vital element in the good development of social skills. This means that in order to acquire and develop social skills, the person has to first develop communication skills, because if we can not communicate adequately and effectively with others, we will never be able to interact adequately at a social level.

If we follow this logic and apply it to AS, we can say that if a person fails in communication she will also fail in socialization, i.e. if a person presents a deficit at the level of communication skills, her social skills will probably also be deficient. An example of this can be seen in the words of Attwood (2009), when he remarks that problems identified at a communicational level with children with AS inhibit their integration in the schoolyard. On the other hand, having an unusual command of linguistic characteristics can produce other social consequences to children with AS. Other children avoid playing with them and when they do, the child with AS is an easy butt of jokes and ridiculed by others due to her particular way of talking.

4. Relation between social cognition and social functioning

So far three main issues have been addressed. Firstly we have explained how AS fits within the spectrum of autism disorders. Secondly, we have analysed the concept of social cognition having explored in detail the most affected components in AS. Finally, social functioning has been examined focusing on social and communication skills that are affected in AS. So far we have AS, social cognition and social functioning as three isolated concepts. What we need to examine now is how the last two (social cognition and social functioning) can be related in AS.

In actual fact, this has been done when the different components of social cognition were examined, since according to Couture et al. (2006) the relation between social functioning and social cognition depends on the specific area of each one of the analyzed constructs. Generally, we can say that there is strong evidence that there is a consistent and clear relation between social cognition and social functioning. Hence, as each of the social cognition components was analysed and deficits identified, the potential implications of those deficits on the life of a person with AS were also mentioned and those implications always have repercussions on a social level.

Therefore, at this point, where the goal is to establish a connection between social cognition and social functioning, it seems relevant to synthesize the information presented thus far in order to present an explanatory model of social functioning impairment in AS that can be caused by the deficits associated with social cognition.

Beginning with the central coherence theory presented in the section dedicated to social perception in AS, we can see that this central coherence is typically weak in AS which means that these people do not pay attention to information as a whole but to detail.

Furthermore, they focus on non-social more than on social information. For example, a person with AS is capable of paying more attention to a living room lamp [non social information] than to all the social information conveyed by the non verbal behaviour of the person she is interacting with, such as facial expression, voice tone, body posture, and more non verbal communication elements.

Given that people with AS prefer to processes details instead of the big picture and that they also prefer non-social rather than socially-relevant information, when she processes the human face, she does not process it in its totality, focusing more on the region of the mouth and paying little attention to the eye region which is the part of the face that transmits the richest information in terms of emotional expression. Through this, we can again see the difficulty felt by these persons in emotional processing, namely on recognizing emotions. In its turn, this influences theory of mind, i.e., if the person with AS cannot recognize emotions in others, this will also present difficulties in attributing mental states to others.

This happens because if the person with AS does not attend to socially relevant information that is transmitting emotional states, she will not be able to perceive what the other person is feeling or thinking. When this occurs, the person with AS feels „lost", because she cannot understand or interpret what is being transmitted, and does not know how to respond or react in a world that is unknown and difficult to understanding. Feeling 'lost in the social world', it is more than natural that the person with AS presents difficulties on a communicational level. She can use verbal language, but fails in other aspects of communication. Taking an example, if the person with AS cannot infer and attribute mental states to others, she will not be able to maintain adequate communication with other people, because she has difficulty in knowing what she should say or do in front of her interlocutors. This leads to communication that is either inadequate or undesirable. In turn, these difficulties in communication will reverberate in social maladjustment. This means that the person with AS, conscious of their difficulties in understanding people and social situations and aware of their inability to communicate and to appropriately interact with others, avoids social contact and social relations, preferring to be in their own world, where everything is always the same, where change and unpredictability do not occur and where everything always seems to be easy. When disconnecting from the world that involves them and shutting themselves into their world, people with AS have more time to focus on their themes of interest and feel better because in their world there are predictable patterns and routines to follow that help in their daily routines.

5. Relationship between Asperger syndrome and alexithymia

The term "alexithymia" was coined by Sifneos in 1972. It is derived from the Greek, with *alexi* meaning "no words" and *thymia* meaning "mood or emotion." Patients with alexithymia have great difficulty or are unable to describe their feelings and can have problems making sophisticated differentiation of one feeling from another. Their communicative style shows markedly reduced or absent symbolic thinking (Taylor, 1984, as cited in Fitzgerald & Molyneux, 2004). As pointed out by Warnes (1986, as cited in Fitzgerald & Molyneux, 2004), these persons "lack the capacity for introspection", they are preoccupied with the "minute detail of external events (...) and are unable to make connections between events, affective arousal and somatic response". Nonverbally, they are "stiff and wooden". They are "mechanical in their object relations". All of these features also fit descriptions of AS, in which the main difficulties are understanding one's own and others' emotions, having problems expressing oneself with nonverbal behavior and in reading that of others. They also have difficulty with "theory of mind" and in predicting the cognitions of others. Their imagination is limited. They tend to have a preoccupation with factual information and are strong in areas such as mathematics, engineering, and computers but can have significant problems with interpersonal relationships. Based on the features of patients with alexithymia and of those with AS, Fitzgerald & Molyneux (2004) defend that, from a clinical perspective, a diagnosis of AS should be considered in patients with alexithymia. According to Fitzgerald & Belgrove (2006) there is significant overlap between alexithymia and AS in various aspects, like cognitive problems, problems with social relationships, speech and language problems, and non-verbal behavior, that is why they emphasise the importance of considering AS in differential diagnosis when psychiatrists are making a diagnosis of Alexithymia.

On the other hand, Hill & Berthoz (2006) suggest that people with AS are likely to show symptoms of alexithymia. This position is sustain by some studies made by these investigators, that report that not all of the persons with AS can be categorised as alexithymic according to their responses to the TAS-20 - Toronto Alexithymia Scale (Bagby, Parker, & Taylor, 1994), that is one the most utilized instruments to measure Alexithymia. Defending this same position, Paula-Pérez et al. (2010) says that clinical experience and research have confirmed that Alexithymia can be recognized in the skills and profile of people with AS.

Silani et al. (2008) examined the inability to identify and distinguish one's own feelings through the use of alexithymia and empathy questionnaires in individuals with AS, compared with matched controls. They have found that the groups differed significantly on both alexithymia and empathy questionnaires, what means that people with AS have higher levels of Alexithymia as well as a lack of empathy. This study also shows that Alexithymia and lack of empathy were correlated, indicating a link between understanding one's own and others' emotions.

Although being two different disorders, AS and Alexithymia present similarities, especially at social cognition levels, with huge impairments in emotional processing and in theory of mind. In our opinion, both diagnoses should exist, because AS is a more complex disorder than Alexithymia. Alexithymia can be present in cases of AS, but not all cases of Alexithymia can be diagnosed with AS. So, it is important to have a profound knowledge about these two clinical conditions when clinicians are about to make a diagnoses.

As mentioned by Fitzgerald & Molyneux (2004), there are two important aspects to future studies in this area. One is to investigate directly the relationship between symptoms of alexithymia and autism spectrum disorders, where Asperger syndrome is included, at the behavioural and cognitive levels. The second is to compare directly individuals with ASD who are/are not alexithymic on their behavioural performance on emotion processing tasks as well as in terms of their neural activity.

6. Conclusion

The main conclusions of this work are the following: AS is a developmental disorder characterized by impairments both in social cognition and in social functioning. Social cognition is a complex construct and includes various components. Three of them have been widely studied in AS, namely emotional processing, theory of mind and social perception and the majority of studies reach the same conclusion: people with AS present deficits in all three areas. These deficits seem to have repercussions on a social level, affecting the social functioning of these persons. Hence these people are unable to interpret the emotions of others, infer mental states, consider other people's perspectives and pay attention to relevant social information. Furthermore, they feel lost in the social world because so impaired they are unable to react in social situations and to establish adequate social interactions in a complex world, that is dictated by social rules, that are hard for them to learn. Given this difficulty in learning social rules, it is very difficult for people with AS to learn and acquire social and communication skills, and this is why these skills are so impaired. Social cognition can be a mediator between non social cognition and social functioning, i.e. we believe that people with AS that present good cognitive capabilities but show difficulties in social cognition, can be functioning in a maladjusted way due to their deficit in social cognition components. If we follow this line of thought, we can predict that if we intervene in social cognition for persons with good cognitive abilities, i.e. in persons with AS, we can be contributing to improving social cognition, and expect to see improvements reverberating in the social functioning of these persons. Since interventions aiming to train social skills are not easily suited to persons with AS, our suggestion for future research is to create programs to work and develop social cognition skills, because if social cognition deficits are the basis of social functioning deficits, we think that if we train and develop social cognition skills, this will have repercussions on the social functioning of these persons and improve their social skills. There is one program that has been developed to this end and that has proven feasible in a pilot study with adults with high functioning autism. This is, the Social Cognition and Interaction Training for Adults with high functioning autism [SCIT-A] (Turner-Brown et al., 2008). Therefore, in future studies, this program and other programs targeting social cognition components should be created and administered to test their feasibility and efficacy in improving social cognition deficits in persons with AS, and to test if improvements in social cognition have repercussions on social functioning improving social and communication skills as well.

7. Acknowledgment

This work was supported by the Ministry of Education and Science of Spain (grant number PSI2009-09421).

8. References

Adams, C., Green, J., Gilchrist, A., & Cox, A. (2002). Conversational behaviour of children with Asperger syndrome and conduct disorder. *Journal of Child Psychology and Psychiatry*, 43, 679-690.

American Psychiatric Association (APA). (2002). *Manual de Diagnóstico e Estatística das Perturbações Mentais* (4ª ed., revisão de texto). Lisboa: Climepsi Editores.

American Psychiatric Association (APA). (2010). Proposed Revision: 299.80 Asperger's Disorder, In: *American Psychiatric Association DSM-5 Development*, 10.07.2011, Available from:
http://www.dsm5.org/ProposedRevisions/Pages/proposedrevision.aspx?rid=97#

Attwood, T. (2009). *Guía del síndrome de Asperger*. Barcelona: Ediciones Paidós Ibérica, S.A.

Bagby, R., Taylor, G., & Parker, J. (1994). The twenty item Toronto Alexithymia Scale-II Convergent, discriminant, and concurrent validity. *Journal of Psychosomatic Research*, 38, 33–40.

Baron-Cohen, S. (1995). *Mind blindness: An essay on autism and theory of mind*. Cambridge: MIT Press.

Baron-Cohen, S. (2001). Theory of mind and autism: a review. *Special Issue of the International Review of Mental Retardation*, 23, 3-24.

Baron-Cohen, S., Spitz, A., & Cross, P. (1993). Can children with autism recognize surprise? *Cognition and Emotion*, 7, 507-516.

Baron-Cohen, S., Jolliffe, T., Mortimore, C., & Robertson, M. (1997a). Another advanced test of theory of mind: Evidence from very high functioning adults with autism or Asperger syndrome. *Journal of Child Psychology and Psychiatry*, 38, 813-822.

Baron-Cohen, S., Wheelwright, S., & Jolliffe, T. (1997b). Is there a "language of the eyes"? Evidence from normal adults and adults with autism or Asperger syndrome. *Visual Cognition*, 4, 311-331.

Baron-Cohen, S., O'Riordan, M., Stone, V., Jones, R., & Plaisted, K. (1999). Recognition of Faux Pas by Normally Developing Children and Children with Asperger Syndrome or High-Functioning Autism. *Journal of Autism and Developmental Disorders*, 29, 407-418.

Baron-Cohen, S., Wheelwright, S., Spong, A., Scachill, V. L., & Lawson, J. (2001). Are intuitive physics and intuitive psychology independent? A test with children with Asperger syndrome. Journal of Developmental and Learning Disorders, 5, 47-78.

Barthélemy, C., Fuentes, J., Van der Gaag, R., & Visconti, P. (2000). *Descrição do Autismo* (documento oficial da Associação Internacional Autisme-Europe). Lisboa: Associação Portuguesa para Protecção aos Deficientes Autistas.

Bassili, J. N. (1979). Emotion recognition: The role of facial movement and the relative importance of upper and lower areas of the face. *Journal of Personality and Social Psychology, 37*, 2049-2058.

Bolton, R. (1979). *People skills: How to assert yourself, listen to others and resolve conflicts*. New York: Simon & Schuster.

Boucher, J., Lewis, V., & Collis, G. M. (2000). Voice processing abilities in children with autism, children with specific language impairments and young typically developing children. *Journal of Child Psychology and Psychiatry and Allied Disciplines, 41*, 847-857.

Bowler, D. M. (1992). Theory of mind in Asperger syndrome. *Journal of Child Psychology and Psychiatry, 33*, 877-895.

Brothers, L. (1990). The social brain: A project for integrating primate behaviour and neurophysiology in new domain. *Concepts in Neuroscience, 1*, 27-61

Calder, A. J., Young, A. W., Keane, J., & Dean, M. (2000). Configural information in facial perception. *Journal of Experimental Psychology: Human Perception and Performance, 26*, 527-551.

Capps, L., Yirmiya, N., & Sigman, M. (1992). Understanding of simple and complex emotions in non-retarded children with autism. *Journal of Child Psychology and Psychiatry, 33*, 1169-1182.

Celani, G., Battacchi, M. W., & Arcidiacono, L. (1999). The understanding of the emotional meaning of facial expressions in people with autism. *Journal of Autism and Developmental Disorders, 29*, 57-66.

Chawarska, K., & Shic, F. (2009). Looking but not seeing: Atypical visual scanning and recognition of faces in 2 and 4-year-old children with autism spectrum disorder. *Journal of Autism and Developmental Disorders, 39*, 1663-1672.

Couture, S., Penn, D., & Roberts, D. (2006). The functional significance of social cognition in schizophrenia: a review. *Schizophrenia Bulletin, 32*, 44-63.

Deruelle, C., Rondan, C., Gepner, B., & Tardif, C. (2004). Spatial frequency and face processing in children with autism and Asperger syndrome. *Journal of Autism and Developmental Disorders, 34*, 199-210.

Fine, C., Lumsden, J., & Blair, R. J. (2001). Dissociation between theory of mind and executive functions in a patient early left amygdale damage. *Brain Journal of Neurology, 124*, 287-298.

Fiske, A. P. (1992). The four elementary forms of sociability : Framework for a unified theory of social relations. *Psychological review, 99*, 689-723.

Fitzgerald, M., & Bellgrove, M. (2006). Letter to the Editor: The overlap between alexithymia and Asperger's syndrome. *Journal of Autism and Developmental Disorders, 36*, 573-576.

Fitzgerald, M., & Molyneux, G. (2004). Letters to Editor: Overlap between alexithymia and Asperger's syndrome. *American Journal of Psychiatry, 161*, 2134-2135.

Freeth, M., Chapman, P., Ropar, D., & Mitchell, P. (2010). Do gaze cues in complex scenes capture and direct the attention of high-functioning adolescents with ASD?

Evidence from eye-tracking. *Journal of Autism and Developmental Disorders*, 40, 534-547.

Frith, U. (2006). *Autismo: Hacia una explicación del enigma (2ª ed.)*. Madrid: Alianza Editorial. (Original work published 1989)

Frith, U., & Happé, F. (1994). Autism: Beyond "theory and mind". *Cognition*, 50, 115-132.

Gillberg, C. (1991). Clinical and neurobiological aspects os Asperger syndrome in six family Studies. In U. Frith (Ed.), *Autism and Asperger syndrome*. Cambridge: Cambridge University Press.

Gillberg, C., & Billstedt, E. (2000). Autism and Asperger syndrome: coexistence with other clinical disorders. *Acta Psychiatrica Scandinavica*, 102, 321-330.

Golan, O., Baron-Cohen, S., & Hill, J. (2006). The Cambridge Mindreading (CAM) face-voice battery: Testing complex emotion recognition in adults with and without Asperger syndrome. *Journal of Autism and Developmental Disorder*, 36, 169-183.

Golan, O., Baron-Cohen, S., & Golan, Y. (2008). The 'reading the mind in films' task (child version): Complex emotion and mental state recognition in children with and without autism spectrum conditions. *Journal of Autism and Developmental Disorder*, 38, 1534-1541.

Grandin, T. (1995). *Thinking in pictures and other reports from my life with autism*. New York: Doubleday.

Grandin, T. (1999). *Visual thinking of a person with autism*. Arlington, TX: Future Horizons, Inc.

Grandin, T., & Barron, S. (2005). *Unwritten rules of social relationships: Decoding social mysteries through the unique perspectives of autism*. Arlington, TX: Future Horizons, Inc.

Grossman, J. B., Klin, A., Carter, A. S., & Volkmar, F. R. (2000). Verbal bias in recognition of facial emotion in children with Asperger syndrome. *Journal of Child Psychology and Psychiatry and Allied Disciplines*, 41, 369-379.

Happé, F. (1993). Communicative competence and theory of mind in autism: a test of relevance theory. *Cognition*, 48, 101-119.

Happé, F. (1994). An advanced test of theory of mind: Understanding of story character's thoughts and feelings by able autistic, mentally handicapped, and normal children and adults. *Journal of Autism and Developmental Disorders*, 24, 129-154.

Happé, F. (1995). The role of age and verbal ability in the theory of mind task performance of subjects with autism. *Child Development*, 66, 843-855.

Happé, F., & Frith, U. (2006). The weak coherence account: Detail-focused cognitive style in autism spectrum disorders. *Journal of Autism and Developmental Disorders*, 36, 5-25.

Hill, E. & Berthoz, S. (2006). Response to "Letter to the Editor: The overlap between alexithymia and Asperger's syndrome", Fitzgerald and Bellgrove. *Journal of Autism and Developmental Disorders*, 36, 1143-1145.

Hobson, R. P. (1986a). The autistic child's appraisal of expressions of emotion. *Journal of Child Psychology and Psychiatry*, 27, 321-342.

Hobson, R. P. (1986b). The autistic child's appraisal of expressions of emotion: A further study. *Journal of Child Psychology and Psychiatry*, 27, 671-680.

Horan, W. P., Kern, R. S., Green, M. F., & Penn, D. (2008). Social Cognition Training for Individuals with Schizophrenia: Emerging Evidence. *American Journal of Psychiatric Rehabilitation*, 11, 205-252.

Kalland, N., Moller-Nielsen, A., Callesen, K., Mortensen, E. L., Gottlieb, D., & Smith, L. (2002). A new "advanced" test of theory of mind: Evidence from children and adolescents with Asperger syndrome. *Journal of Child Psychology and Psychiatry*, 43, 517-528.

Kalland, N., Callesen, K., Moller-Nielsen, A., Mortensen, E. L., & Smith, L. (2008). Performance of children and adolescents with Asperger syndrome or high-functoning autism on advanced theory of mind tasks. *Journal of Autism and Developmental Disorders*, 38, 1112-1123.

Kleinman, J., Marciano, P. L., & Ault, R. L. (2001). Advanced theory of mind in high-functioning adults with autismo. *Journal of Autism and Developmental Disorders*, 31, 29-36.

Klin, A. (1991). Young autistic children's listening preferences in regard to speech: A possible characteristic of the symptom of social withdrawal. *Journal of Autism and Developmental Disorders*, 21, 29-42.

Klin, A. (1992). Listening preferences in regard to speech in four children with developmental disabilities. *Journal of Child Psychology and Psychiatry*, 3, 763-769.

Klin, A., & Jones, W. (2008). Altered face scanning and impaired recognition of biological motion in a 15-month-old infant with autism. *Developmental Science*, 11, 40-46.

Klin, A., Jones, W., Schultz, R., Volkmar, F., & Cohen, D. (2002a). Defining and quantifying the social phenotype in autism. *American Journal of Psychiatry*, 159, 895-908.

Klin, A., Jones, W., Schultz, R., Volkmar, F., & Cohen, D. (2002b). Visual fixation patterns during viewing of naturalistic social situations as predictors of social competence in individuals with autism. *Archives of General Psychiatry*, 59, 808-816.

Klin, A., & Volkmar, F. (1997). Autism and the pervasive developmental disorders. In J. Noshpitz (Ed.) *Handbook of child and adolescent psychiatry* (Vol. 1, pp. 536-560). New York: Wiley.

Koning, C. & Magill-Evans, J. (2001). Social and language skills in adolescent boys with Asperger syndrome. *Autism*, 5, 23-36.

Kuusikko, S., Haapsamo, H., Jansson-Verkasalo, E., Hurtig, T., Matilla, M., Ebeling, H., Jussila, K., Bölte, S., & Moilanen, I. (2009). Emotion recognition in children and adolescents with autism spectrum disorders. *Journal of Autism and Developmental Disorders*, 39, 938-945.

Leslie, A. M. (1987). Pretence and representation: The origins of "Theory of mind". *Psychological Review*, 94, 412-426.

Loveland, K. A., Tunali Kotoski, B., Chen, R., & Brelsford, K. A. (1995). Intermodal perception of affect in persons with autism or Down syndrome. *Development and Psychopathology*, 7, 409-418.

MacDonald, H., Rutter, M., Howlin, P., Le Conteur, A., Evered, C., et al. (1989). Recognition and expression of emotional cues by autistic and normal adults. *Journal of Child Psychology and Psychiatry*, 30, 865-877.

Manjiviona, J., & Prior, M. (1999). Neuropsychological profiles of children with Asperger syndrome and autism. *Autism*, 3, 327-356.

Marcondes, D. (2000). Desfazendo mitos sobre a pragmática. *ALCEU*, 1, 38-46.

Mehrabian, A. (1972). *Nonverbal communication*. Chicago: Aldine-Atherton.

Miller, J. N., & Ozonoff, S. (2000). The external validity of Asperger disorder: Lack of evidence from the domain of neuropsychology. *Journal of Abnormal Psychology*, 109, 227-238.

Mongillo, E. A., Irwin, J. R., Whalen, D. H., Klaiman, C., Carter, A. S., & Schultz, R. T. (2008). Audiovisual processing in children with and without autism spectrum disorders. *Journal of Autism and Developmental Disorders*, 38, 1349-1358.

Ozonoff, S., Pennington, B.F., & Rogers, S. (1991). Executive function deficits in high-functioning autistic individuals: Relationship to theory of mind. *Journal of Child Psychology and Psychiatry*, 32, 1081-1105.

Patrick, N. J. (2008). *Social skills for teenagers and adults with Asperger syndrome*. London: Jessica Kingsley Publishers.

Paul, R., Augustyn, A., Klin, A., & Volkmar, F. (2005). Perception and production of prosody by speakers with autism spectrum disorders. *Journal of Autism and Developmental Disorders*, 35, 205-220.

Paul, R., & Landa, R. (2008). Communication in Asperger syndrome. In A. Klin, S. Sparrow, & F. Volkmar (Eds.), *Asperger syndrome* (2nd ed.). New York: Guildford Press.

Paul, R., & Sutherland, D. (2003). Asperger syndrome: the role of the speech-language pathologists in schools. *Perspectives on Language, Learning and Education*, 10, 9-15.

Paula-Pérez, I., Martos-Pérez, J., & Llorente-Comí, M. (2010). Alexithymia and Asperger syndrome. *Revue Neurologique*, 50, S85-S90.

Pelphrey, K. A., Sasson, N. J., Reznick, J., Paul, G., Goldman, B. D., & Piven, J. (2002). Visual scanning of faces in autism. *Journal of Autism and Developmental Disorders*, 32, 249-261.

Ponnet, K. S., Roeyers, H., Buyesse, A., De Clercq, A., & Van der Heyden, E. (2004). Advanced mind-reading in adults with Asperger syndrome. *Autism*, 8, 249-266.

Ritvo, E., & Freeman, B. (1978). National Society for Autistic Children definition of the syndrome of autism. *Journal of Autism and Developmental Disorders*, 8, 162-169.

Ruiz-Ruiz, J. C., García-Ferrer, S. & Fuentes-Durá, I. (2006). La relevancia de la cognición social en la esquizofrenia. *Apuntes de Psicología*, 24, 137-155.

Rutherford, M. D., Baron-Cohen, S., & Wheelwright, S. (2002). Reading the mind in the voice: A study with normal adults and adults with Asperger syndrome and high-functioning autism. *Journal of Autism and Developmental Disorders*, 32, 189-194.

Shamay-Tsoory, S. G. (2008). Recognition of 'fortune of others' emotions in Asperger syndrome and high functioning autism. *Journal of Autism and Developmental Disorders*, 38, 1451-1461.

Sheppard, E., Ropar, D., Underwood, G., & Van Loon, E. (2010). Brief report: Driving hazard perception in autism. *Journal of Autism and Developmental Disorders*, 40, 504-508.

Shriberg, L., Paul, R., McSweeney, J., & Klin, A. (2001). Speech and prosody characteristics of adolescents and adults with high-functioning autism and Asperger syndrome. *Journal of Speech, Language and Hearing Research*, 44, 1097-1115.

Sicile-Kira, C. (2006). *Adolescents on the autism spectrum: A parent's guide to the cognitive, social, physical and transition needs of teenagers with autism spectrum disorders*. New York: Penguin Group.

Sicile-Kira, C. (2008). *Autism life skills: From communication and safety to self-esteem and more*. New York: Penguin Group.

Silani, G., Bird, G., Brindley, R., Singer, T., Frith, C., & Frith, U. (2008). Levels of emotional awareness and autism: An fmRI study. *Social Neuroscience*, 3, 97-112.

Speer, L. L., Cook, A. E., McMahon, W. M., & Clark, E. (2007). Face processing in children with autism: Effects of stimulus contents and type. *Autism*, 11, 265-277.

Spek, A. A., Scholte, E. M., & Berckelaer-Onnes, I. A. (2010). Theory of mind in adults with HFA and Asperger syndrome. *Journal of Autism and Developmental Disorder*, 40, 280-289.

Spezio, M. L., Adolphs, R., Hurley, R. S. E., & Piven, J. (2007). Abnormal use of facial information in high-functioning autism. *Journal of Autism and Developmental Disorder*, 37, 929-939.

Striano, T., & Reid, V. (2009). *Social Cognition: Development, Neuroscience and Autism*. Oxford: Wiley-BlackWell.

Tager-Flusberg, H., Paul, R., & Lord, C. (2005). Language and communication in autism. In F. Volkmar, R. Paul, A. Klin, & D. Cohen (Eds.), *Handbook of autism and pervasive developmental disorders* (3rd ed., Vol. 1, pp. 335-364). New York: Wiley.

Turner-Brown, L., Perry, T. D., Dichter, G. S., Bodfish, J. W., & Penn, D. L. (2008). Brief report: Feasibility of social cognition and interaction training for adults with high functioning autism. *Journal of Autism and Developmental Disorders*, 38, 1777-1784.

Watzlawick, P., Beavin, J., & Jackson, D. (1967). *Pragmatics of Human Communication*. New York : W. W. Norton.

Windle, R., & Warren, S. (1999). *Communication Skills*. In: *Center for Appropriate Dispute Resolution in Special Education [CADRE]*, 15.July.2010, Available from: http//www.directionservice.org/cadre/contents.cfm

Yirmiya, N., Sigman, M. D., Kasari, C., & Mundy, P. (1992). Empathy and cognition in high-functioning children with autism

8

Suicidal Cut Throat Injuries: Management Modalities

Adeyi A. Adoga

Senior Lecturer/Consultant Ear, Nose, Throat, Head and Neck Surgeon
Department of Ear, Nose, Throat/ Head and Neck Surgery
University of Jos and Jos University Teaching Hospital
Nigeria

1. Introduction

Suicide is defined as the act of taking one's life. This self destructive act constitutes an individual intentionally or ambivalently taking his or her own life.

Suicidal behavior is any deliberate action with potentially life-threatening consequences, such as taking a drug overdose or deliberately crashing a car.

Oftentimes suicide is committed by individuals suffering from a mental illness; therefore, it can be used as an index of mental ill health in a community.

Several forms of suicidal behavior exists which fall within the self destructive spectrum. These include;

Suicide attempt: This involves a serious act, such as inflicting self injury and some other person accidentally intervening. Without the accidental discovery, death of the individual would occur.

Suicide gesture: This is when an individual undertakes an unusual but not fatal behavior as a cry for help or to get attention.

Suicide gamble: This is inflicting self injury knowing that family members or other persons will be home in time to discover and save them.

Suicide equivalent: In this situation an individual does not attempt suicide. Instead, he or she uses behavior to get some of the reactions their suicide would have caused. For example, an adolescent boy runs away from home. He wants to see how his parents respond to his absence from home. He wants to know if they care, if they are sorry for the way that they have been treating him. This can be seen as an indirect cry for help.

There are various ways of executing suicide ranging from ingestion of fatal drug dosages to slitting one's wrists, hanging by the neck to cutting of the throat. Cut throat injuries may be homicidal or suicidal and they are potentially life threatening injuries because of the many vital structures in the neck which may be affected leading to sever hemorrhage, air embolism or respiratory obstruction and death. Therefore, prompt and adequate intervention is required following a cut throat injury from an attempted suicide to save a patient. This chapter aims to discuss the management modalities available for cut throat injuries with suicide as the motivating factor.

2. Epidemiology

Suicide is one of the ten leading causes of death in the world with about one million deaths recorded annually [1]. The incidence and pattern of suicide varies from one geographical location to the other because religious, cultural and social values play an important role in its occurrence.

In the United States it is the eleventh leading cause of death[2]. An alarming estimated 700,000 people worldwide attempt suicide annually [3].

Overall, 2.9 percent of the adult population attempts suicide and the suicide rate in the general population over a lifetime period of 70 years is about 1 percent [4, 5]. Studies of suicide attempters suggest that one percent to two percent complete suicide within a year after the initial attempt, with another one percent committing suicide in each following year[6].

Suicides in Ife, western Nigeria were found to be 0.4 per 100,000 population in 2001 with a higher incidence in males with a male to female ratio of 3.6 to 1. The majority of the victims were in the third decade of life[7].

Men commit suicide far more frequently than women. In a study in the United States in 2004, the suicide rate for men was 18.0 per 100,000 population and 4.5 per 100,000 populations for women [8]. However, women make far more suicidal attempts than men.

The rate increases with age with a major peak in adolescents and young infants. Interestingly however, geriatric suicide is becoming prevalent with individuals older than 65 years having the highest rate of suicide [2].

Suicides occurring from cut throat injuries are rarely reported in the medical literature but they do occur. They may occur either in isolation or as part of multiple injuries in a poly-traumatized patient.

3. Risk factors

The risk factors for suicide are classified as proximal or distal and within these broad groups as either;
1.   Mental illness
2.   Socio-demographic
3.   Familial
4.   Biological
5.   Situational (life experiences) risk factors.

Mental illnesses are the strongest predictors of suicide [1]. Suicide occurs 20.4 times more frequently in individuals with major depression than the general population [9]. Older people who are depressed are also more at risk of committing suicide than younger depressed individuals [4].

The prevalence of major depressive disorder in western industrialized nations is 2.3 percent to 3.2 percent for men and 4.5 percent to 9.3 percent for women. The lifetime risk of depression ranges from 7 to 12 percent for men and 20 percent to 25 percent for women. Studies indicate that the risk of depression is not related to race, education, or income [5].

In a 5 year study in New Zealand, of 302 individuals making medically serious suicide attempts, 67 percent died by suicide and 37 percent made at least one fatal attempt. Hence, there is a need for enhanced follow-up, treatment and surveillance of any individual making suicide attempts [10].

Other mental illnesses linked with suicide are schizophrenia, anxiety disorders, post-traumatic stress disorder, delirium, dementia and substance abuse.

A positive family history is also regarded as a predictive factor therefore careful assessment of family history of mental illnesses and suicide should also be a routine aspect of patient evaluation.

Unemployment can act as a stressor leading to suicide [11] with studies suggesting an increase in the parasuicide and suicide rates among unemployed individuals than in the general population [12]. This is more so for the male who is the breadwinner of the family in many societies. He can get frustrated when not able to meet family needs and want to take his own life [13]. It is a known fact that the suicide rate among non-waged workers is significantly higher than that of waged workers [14].

Socio-demographic factors linked to suicide are sex, type of occupation, alcohol consumption and the availability of a weapon such as a rope, knife or gun. Others are religion, ethnicity, and even seasons. The regions of the world with long, dark winter seasons such as Scandinavia and parts of Alaska like Nome are known to have higher suicide rates.

Some life events are also linked with the act of committing suicide for example a child who witnesses a family member committing suicide may later make similar attempts and kill himself or herself.

Scientists believe that the interplay of several factors which lead to depression is very complex. Family studies have shown that 20 to 50 percent of children and adolescents who experience depression have a positive family history of depression [15, 16, 17, 18] and children of depressed parents are three times more likely to experience a depressive disorder [19]. They are also more vulnerable to other mental and somatic disorders [20]. It is however not clear if depressed parents create an environment that increases the chances of a mental disorder developing in their children. Like other mental illnesses, depression is probably caused by a combination of biological, environmental and social factors as mentioned above. The exact causes are however not yet known. Scientists have thought for a long time that low brain levels of neurotransmitters like serotonin, dopamine and norepinephrine was responsible for depression.

There can be underlying physical reasons for severe depression in certain individuals. For example, individuals diagnosed with a terminal illness, or those living with a long term physical disability, especially if accompanied by pain that is never likely to go away. It can be much harder to treat depression for individuals in this category, as the underlying causes are physical issues that cannot be cured. That is not to say though that even individuals such as this cannot find a motivating reason for living. Table 1 below shows some medical conditions associated with an increased risk of suicide. Suicide attempters are noted to have higher rates of comorbid mental illnesses and individuals who have attempted suicide in the past also have an increased chance of future suicidal behavior.

The incidence and pattern of suicide varies from country to country. Hanging, poisoning and drowning are the commonest methods of committing suicide in some regions of the world. Other not so common methods of committing suicide documented in the literature include;

1. Suffocation.
2. Electrocution.
3. Jumping from a height.
4. Vehicular impact.
5. Immolation.
6. Hypothermia.

7. Starvation (apocarteresis).
8. Dehydration.
9. Firearms.
10. 'belly slitting' a rather interesting method also referred to as *Seppuku*.

Cancer	Chronic pain	Hypertension
HIV/AIDS	Chronic renal failure	Epilepsy
Multiple sclerosis	Spinal cord injuries	Peptic ulcer disease
Cardiopulmonary disease	Huntington's chorea	Rheumatoid arthritis
Organic brain syndromes	Head injury	Cushing's syndrome

Table 1. Medical conditions associated with increased risk of suicide

Suicide by means of cut throat is either rare as reported by some or common as reported by other researchers. The paucity of reports from some parts of the world like Nigeria may be because these injuries are rare or underreported [13]. Throat-cutting is not indigenous to Nigeria or any other country for that matter. The mode of committing or attempting suicide depends on the type of weapon available to the individual. From various reports in Nigeria, the commonest method of committing suicide seems to be the ingestion of poisonous materials followed by the use of weapons like the knife and the Dane gun [7, 21, 22].

The scope of this chapter does not include discussions on the other methods of suicide mentioned above but it is important to note them.

4. Management

Suicide is preventable therefore in many cases swift decisive intervention can prevent an individual from committing it. Intervention is based on the application of risk factors with adequate clinical inquiry.

When suicidal cut throat injuries occur, a multidisciplinary approach is required in the effective management of victims. This requires the close collaboration of the Otorhinolaryngologist, the anesthesiologist and the psychiatrist [23].

The diagnosis is based on anamnestic data, clinical check-up and inspection of the pharynx, larynx, esophagus and contiguous structures to determine the extent of injury.

The neck contains vital structures- neurovascular bundles, larynx, trachea, esophagus and spinal cord etc in a small compartment, therefore these injuries are life threatening and present as emergencies. The injuries are varied and depend on the pattern, site and depth of the cut on the neck.

The severity of the injury is assessed by assigning the injury to areas or zones of the neck. This way, the vital structures affected in the course of injury can be determined. Injuries of the neck are divided into three anatomic zones for the purpose of ease of assessment;

1. Zone l injuries occur at the thoracic inlet. This zone extends from the level of the cricoid cartilage to the clavicles.

2.   Zone ll injuries are those occurring in the region between the cricoid cartilage and the angle of the mandible. Injuries in this zone are the easiest to expose and evaluate.

3.   Zone lll injuries occur between the angle of the mandible and the base of the skull.

Unlike zone ll, zones l and lll are protected by bony structures making zone ll more vulnerable to injuries.

Assessment of these patients begins with the ABCs of resuscitation i.e checking the airway, evaluating the patient's breathing and circulation. Resuscitation of individuals is commenced immediately. When the victims present;

1.   The anesthesiologist secures an uncompromised airway and makes sure the patient is breathing.

2.   The otorhinolaryngologist assesses the injury and surgically repairs the severed tissues with the aim of restoration of breathing, swallowing and phonation.

3.   The psychiatrist provides adequate care and supervision during and after surgical repair of severed tissues.

If the victims present without airway compromise, an assessment of the severed tissues is made and meticulous surgical repair effected in the shortest possible time.

Securing the airway is the first priority in the management of these patients if the airway is unstable or in the presence of edema. The ideal way to establish airway is orotracheal intubation in the awake patient which is followed by the insertion of a tracheostomy tube through the transected portion of the trachea if a transection is present. Some authors have described this approach to be dangerous because it can produce a further damage to the larynx or increasing the chances of inhaling vomitus, blood or secretions [24]. However, a formal tracheostomy can be done in the early phases of presentation to secure the airway and anesthetic gases can be administered via this in order to carry out repair under general anesthesia. Although, in severe airway compromise reports have been made of airway maintenance with endotracheal intubation alone and there have been reports of the effective use of a fibreoptic laryngoscope to intubate the trachea following a cut throat injury [25]. This has reduced the need for tracheostomy and its attendant complications. In the event that the trachea is completely transected, a re-anastomosis of the transected ends of the trachea is done. Most practitioners advocate the use of absorbable suture in achieving this. One or two stainless steel wires can be used in addition to the absorbable sutures to provide strength to the anastomosed tracheal ends. Bryce demonstrates this in his work and to relieve the tension on the anastomosis, he keeps the patient's neck flexed postoperatively for seven to ten days by suturing the chin to the sternum [26]. Sometimes, a segment of the trachea may be badly damaged requiring resection. It is generally agreed that the maximal length of trachea resectable is 7cm and the cut ends of the trachea would require mobilization in the neck in order to achieve anastomosis by a laryngeal release procedure or in addition by splitting the sternum and mobilizing the main stem bronchi [27]. The combination of these three procedures can achieve a mobilization of the trachea for a distance of 7cm. In achieving mobilization of the cervical trachea, the surgeon needs to bear in mind the fact that the blood supply of the trachea is placed laterally from the inferior thyroid artery and the right bronchial artery. Therefore, mobilization should be only in an anterio-posterior plane leaving the lateral fibrous attachment untouched.

Once the airway is secured, the treatment option is timely surgical repair of the severed tissues in order to restore structure and functions. These injuries will involve the soft tissues, neurovascular bundles, cartilage and bones all or in part depending on the magnitude of impact of the cutting agent used. The extent of repair is therefore determined by the extent of injury.

Blood tests (urgent packed cell volume, urea and electrolyte levels), angiography, endoscopy (esophagoscopy, microlaryngoscopy and bronchoscopy) and computerized tomographic (CT) scan helps to determine the extent of injury. Individuals are transfused with whole blood depending on the extent of blood loss. Plain radiography alone is not sufficient to diagnose airway trauma and the additional use of dynamic CT scan of the trachea and larynx and magnetic resonance imaging (MRI) can be very helpful in discovering previously undetected injuries, showing that some of these injuries may not even require surgical intervention. However, adequate airway management should not be delayed by radiologic studies because an apparently stable airway can rapidly progress into an acute airway obstruction [28, 29].

In some environment, late presentation is a common feature due to factors like ignorance and of course poverty which may also invariably be the triggering factor for the suicidal attempt. In the event of late presentation, debridement of infected tissues is also done prior to suturing (Figure 1). Debridement may also mean loss of substantial amounts of tissue to effect simple and proper closure. Ideally, pharyngeal, hypopharyngeal and laryngeal mucosal lacerations should be repaired early because the time elapsed before repair of laryngeal mucosal lacerations has an effect on both airway stenosis and on voice restoration [30]. Soft laryngeal stent may be needed for severely macerated mucosa.

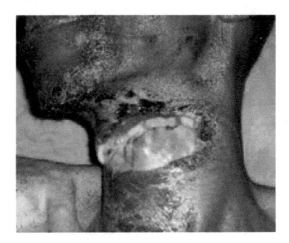

Fig. 1. Infected suicidal cut throat injury at presentation.

A pharyngo-cutaneous fistula must be prevented as much as possible while carrying out pharyngo-hypopharyngeal repair. This requires meticulous approximation of the tissues, use of a nasogastric (NG) tube and avoidance of oral feeding for a period of 7 -10 days. If a pharyngo- cutaneous fistula occurs, NG tube feeding must continue until the fistula closes. If the fistula persists for more than 6 weeks, it may indicate either the presence of a foreign body, wrong surgical technique, malnutrition or a concomitant underlying malignancy especially in the elderly. Such extreme cases may need flap closure using local, regional or distant flaps after excision of the fistula. To avoid the discomfort of inserting an NG tube, the risks of aspiration and the effect of an impinging foreign body at the injury site, Darlong et al have advocated the creation of a feeding jejunostomy which is used to maintain enteral feeding [31]. This involves passing a catheter through the anterior abdominal wall into the jejunal lumen via an intramural tunnel. The catheter is advanced distally to prevent reflux and it is then secured using purse-string suture. Any excess catheter length is removed from the peritoneal cavity until the jejunum lies adjacent to the parietal peritoneum. Interrupted stitches are then used to secure the jejunum in place.

Complications may follow a feeding jejunostomy and should be noted and addressed appropriately. These complications are;

1. Nausea.
2. Diarrhea.
3. Constipation.
4. Abdominal distention.
5. Abdominal cramps.
6. Reflux.
7. Catheter blockage.
8. Pericatheter leakage.
9. Catheter dislodgement.
10. Jejunal perforation.

Tissue injury may be as extensive such as severe laryngeal injuries as to warrant a total laryngectomy.

Careful handling and suturing of the severed tissues usually gives a reasonably good outcome with the restoration of breathing, swallowing and phonation (Figure 2).

Individuals are then weaned off their endotracheal tubes, tracheostomy or NG tubes before discharge.

Mental health intervention is one of the most important parts of managing suicidal cut throat attempts. After suicidal behavior is addressed, any underlying disorders should be treated. Mental disorders like depression, schizophrenia, substance abuse, alcohol dependence should be sought from proper clinical assessment of individuals and treated.

Even following discharge from otorhinolaryngological care, individuals should be closely followed and supervised in other to prevent another suicidal attempt that may actually lead to the death of these individuals. Those who try to commit suicide should be assessed and treated to reduce the risk of future attempts. All suicide attempts and expressions of suicidal intent should be taken seriously regardless of whether the individual has made multiple past attempts of low lethality, regardless of the presence of a suspected personality disorder and even if it has been suggested that the attempt was with the aim to manipulate other people. Sometimes a patient's suicidal gesture will be described as 'attention-seeking'. This term is often used in a derogatory term and is best to avoid this as it is likely to negatively influence an otherwise objective risk assessment.

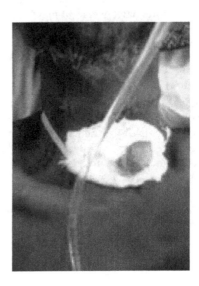

Fig. 2. Repaired cut throat injury.

Some authors are of the opinion that self-harm attempts can be grouped into 'serious suicide attempts' and more impulsive forms of deliberate self-harm. The former is typically associated with severe mental illness, high intended lethality and attempts by the suicide attempter to avoid rescue. The latter is considered a manifestation of personality disorder or acute crisis, where there are impulsive, poorly planned attempts at self harm. This rule of thumb may be misleading, regardless of the potential for death or serious injury in the deliberate self harm category, the rates of completed suicide years after a seemingly minor episode of so called 'deliberate self harm' are significant. This fact is highlighted in a study done in Australia in which 223 patients were followed from 1975 onwards. Of those who had made an attempt at deliberate self harm in the mid 1970's, 4% had completed suicide at 4 years, 4.5% at ten years and 6-7% by 18 years.

The following are important in the assessment of suicide attempters;

1. Building a rapport- These patients may be depressed, embarrassed or guarded; therefore they may be reluctant in volunteering a history. They are relieved and corporative by the unburdening of their troubles rather than being annoyed and offended at them.

2. Taking a psychiatric history- Information regarding the attempt or intent of suicide should be obtained in an open and direct manner without any form of ambiguity. It is helpful to introduce questions regarding the suicide in a sequential manner. It is often

useful to run through the chronological events leading up to, during and after the suicide attempt to assess the level of risk.

Risk assessment is the process of estimating the degree of dangerousness to self and to others and it should be known that the strongest predictor of future dangerousness is past dangerousness [32]. There are two approaches to risk assessment;

- The actuarial assessment.
- The standardized clinical assessment.

The actuarial approach to risk assessment is inferior to a standardized clinical assessment [33] because it provides little more than passive prediction [34]. The apparent superiority of clinical judgment appears to relate to its emphasis upon prevention, rather than prediction. The approach to the acute assessment of dangerousness requires consideration of both "static" and "dynamic" risk factors. Static risk factors are the components of a particular patient's presentation, which are not amenable to intervention, such as age, gender or aspects of a patient's previous history, such as a past history of violent offending. By contrast, dynamic risk factors are those which are potentially changeable to clinical intervention, such as active psychotic symptoms, problematic living circumstances or substance abuse. The value of such an approach is that certain factors amenable to clinical intervention can be identified and implemented, thus potentially reducing risk.

Other factors to consider when taking a psychiatric history are;

a. Events prior to suicide attempt: ask about the following;
    - exposure to significant acute psychosocial stressors or medical problems which may be the precipitating or motivating factors.
    - presence of low mood or symptoms of major illness.
    - feelings of hopelessness.
    - substance abuse.
    - conscious efforts at a preparation for death e.g. finalization of will.
    - onset of suicidal ideation.
    - degree of planning versus impulsivity.
    - the patients perception of the degree of harm to be inflicted on self by the chosen method of suicide.

b. Events at the time of the act of suicide: ask about;
    - the setting at the time of suicide attempt.
    - the presence of stressors.

c. Events following the suicidal attempt:
    - is the patient sad or glad that he is alive following suicide attempt?
    - any exhibition of remorse about the attempt?
    - did the patient call for help after the attempt?
    - is the patient still in possession of the object used in the attempted suicide?
    - is the patient willing to accept treatment?
    - presence of ongoing intents.
    - patients ongoing plans for the future.
    - avalaibility of support in the community for the patient.
    - has the attempt at suicide helped the patient in the release of his/her frustrations?

d. Past psychiatric history:

- previous suicide attempts and all the events that occurred at the time.
- presence or absence of a diagnosed mental illness or personality disorders.

e.   Collateral history:

This is obtained from the past medical files, family members and friends. In this case issues of privacy and confidentiality must be weighed against the level of risk.

5. Medical and physical assessment

Thorough physical assessment of the patient is done by the medical staff. Assessment of the patient's cognitive functions may be important here. Sedatives may be given to reduce the patient's distress or risk of harmful behavior.

It is important that the patient is medically stable before being transferred to the psychiatric ward.

The aim of psychiatric management is to treat the condition that may have led to suicide attempt. Irrespective of the condition acting as trigger for suicide, psychosocial interventions play an important role in the management of these patients. Table 2 below shows some pharmacological agents used in the treatment of these conditions.

Risk factors	Pharmacological agents
Schizophrenia	Clozapine
Bipolar disorder	Sodium valproate, Carbamazepine, Lamotrigine, Gabapetin, Lithium, (these are used as mood stabilizers)
Psychosis	Haloperidol, Resperidone, Flupenthixol
Major depression	Tricyclic antidepressants (TCAs), Selective serotonin reuptake inhibitors (SSRIs)

Table 2. Pharmacological agents used in the treatment of conditions associated with suicide.

6. Management of complications

Surgical repair can be complicated by the long term morbidity of laryngo-tracheal stenosis and pharyngocutaneous fistula [35, 36]. These follow grossly damaged and infected laryngotracheal structures in a cut throat injury especially when poorly managed ab initio. Proper initial management and early repair of the cut throat injury will prevent the development of these complications. Two methods of treatment can be employed for laryngotracheal stenosis- endoscopic and open surgery. Open surgery is the treatment of choice because in the long term it provides a better success rate and functional results.

However, if a contraindication exists to an external approach, laser assisted endoscopy with stenting can also provide good palliative results [37].

7. Prevention

Suicide attempts and threats should always be taken seriously. About one-third of people who attempt suicide will repeat the attempt within 1 year, and about 10% of those who threaten or attempt suicide eventually do kill themselves.

Individuals who are suicidal have a number of characteristics, including the following:

- A preoccupation with death or even stating the desire to harm themselves.
- A sense of isolation and withdrawal from friends and family.
- Anhedonia: distraction and lacking the sense of humor.
- Performing self-destructive behaviors, such as drinking alcohol or substance abuse.
- Focusing on the past: dwelling in past losses and defeats and anticipate no future. They voice the notion that others and the world would be better off without them.
- They are haunted and dominated by hopelessness and helplessness.

When an individual is noted with these symptoms mental health care should be sought immediately. Dismissing the person's behavior as attention-seeking can have devastating consequences.

It is important to note that not all individuals who are exposed to risk factors develop suicidal behaviors. It therefore means that there are certain protective factors that act to mitigate the effects of exposure of individuals to risk factors. These protective factors act to counter the adverse effects or moderate the impact of risk factors and they are classed as follows;

1. Individual attributes: These include
   a. Cognitive abilities such as Intelligence Quotient (IQ) scores and executive functioning skills.
   b. Temperament control.
   c. Personality e.g. adaptability.
   d. Self regulation skills such as the control of impulsive behavior.
   e. Self perceptions of competence/Self esteem.
   f. A positive outlook on life.
2. Relationships:
   a. Relationships with competent adults e.g. parents, mentors and other family members.
   b. Interaction with members of a social peer group.
3. Community resources and societal opportunities:
   a. Good and proper schools.
   b. Connections with social and societal organizations such as religious groups.
   c. A good and qualitative neighborhood.
   d. Proper health care and social amenities.

8. Summary/Conclusion

Suicide is preventable and identifying the risk factors with rapid and decisive interventions can save lives.

Even as screening and the treatment of mental disorders is important, ways must also be found to identify the many people without mental disorders who are at risk of suicidal behaviors.

9. References

[1] Nock MK, Hwang I, Sampson N, et al: Cross-National Analysis of the Associations among Mental Disorders and Suicidal Behavior: Findings from the WHO World Mental Health Surveys. PLoS Med 2009, 6(8): e1000123.

[2] Suicide in the U.S.: Statistics and Prevention. National Institute of Mental Health. Available at:
http://www.nimh.nih.gov/health/publications/suicide-in-the-us-statistics-and-prevention.shtml. Accessed Sept 15, 2008.

[3] Comer RJ. Suicide. In: *Abnormal Psychology.* 6th ed. New York: Worth Publishers; 2007:278-307.

[4] D. C. Clark, "Rational Suicide and People with Terminal Conditions or Disabilities," Issues in Law and Medicine 8 (1992):147-66.

[5] Depression Guideline Panel, Depression in Primary Care, vol. 1, Detection and Diagnosis, Clinical Practice Guideline, no. 5, AHCPR pub. no. 93-0550 (Rockville, Md.: U. S. Department of Health and Human Services, Public Health Sec, Agency for Health Care Policy and Research, April 1993), 36.

[6] G. M. Asnis et al., "Suicidal Behaviors in Adult Psychiatric Outpatients, I: Description and Prevalence," American Journal of Psychiatry 150 (1993): 108-12.

[7] Nwosu SO, Odesanmi WO. Pattern of suicides in Ile-Ife, Nigeria. West Afr J Med. 2001; 20(3): 259-62.

[8] Suicides in the United States 2004. From the CDC WISQARS website. Available at:
http://www.cdc.gov/ncipc/wisqars/default.htm.

[9] Terra JL: Suicide risk and depression. Rev Prat 2008, 58(4):385-8.

[10] Beautrais AL: Further suicidal behavior among medically serious suicide attempters. Suicide Life Threat Behav 2004, 34(1):1-11.

[11] Shah A, Bhandarkar R: Cross-national study of the correlation of general population suicide rates with unemployment rates. Psychol Rep 2008, 103(3):793-6.

[12] Platt S: Unemployment and suicidal behavior: a review of the literature. Soc Sci Med 1984, 19(2):93-115.

[13] Adoga AA, Ma'an ND, Embu HY, Obindo JT Management of suicidal cut throat injuries in a developing nation: three case reports. Cases Journal 2010; 3:65.

[14] Gallagher LM, Kliem C, Beautrais AL, Stallones L: Suicide and occupation in New Zealand, 2001-2005. Int J Occup Environ Health 2008, 14(1):45-50.

[15] Birmaher B, Ryan ND, Williamson DE, Brent DA, Kaufman J. Childhood and adolescentdepression: A review of the past 10 years. Part ll. J Am Acad Child Adolesc Psychiatry. 1996,35; 1575-1583.

[16] Kovacs M, Devlin B, Pollack M, Richards C, Mukerji P. A controlled family history study of childhood-onset depressive disorder. Arch Gen Psychiatry. 1997, 54; 613-623.

[17] Puig-Antich J, Goetz D, Davies M, Kaplan T, Davies S, Ryan ND. A controlled family history study of prepubertal major depressive disorder. Arch Gen Psychiatry. 1989, 54; 1417-1426.

[18] Todd RD, Neuman R, Geller B, Fox LW, Hickok J. Genetic studies of affective disorders: should we be starting with childhood onset probands? J Am Acad child AdolesC Psychiatry. 1993, 32; 1164-1171.

[19] Williamson DE, Ryan ND, Birmaher B, Dahl RE, Kaufman J, Rao U, Puig-Antich J. A case –controlled family history study of depression in adolescents. J Am Acad child Adolesc Psychiatry. 1995, 34: 1596-1607.

[20] Dowrey G, Coyne JC. Children of depressed parents: An integrative review. Psychological Bulletin. 1990, 108: 50-76.

[21] Ogunleye AO, Nwaorgu GB, Grandawa H. Corrosive oesophagitis in Nigeria: clinical spectrums and implications. Trop Doct. 2002;32(2):78-80.

[22] Okulate GT. Suicide attempts in a Nigerian military setting. East Afr J Med. 2001; 78(9): 493-6.

[23] Herzog M, Hoppe F, Baier G, Dieler R: Injuries of the head and neck in suicidal intention. Laryngorhinootologie 2005, 84(3):176-81

[24] Schaefer SD, Close LG. Acute management of laryngeal trauma. Update. Ann Otol Rhinol Laryngol. 1989; 98: 98-104.

[25] Venkatachalam SG, Palaniswamy Selvaraj DA, Rangarajan M, Mani K, Palanivelu C: An unusual case of penetrating tracheal ("cut throat") injury due to chain snatching: the ideal airway management. Indian J Crit Care Med 2007, 11(3): 151-4.

[26] Bryce DP. The surgical management of laryngotracheal injury. J Laryngol Otol. 1972; 86: 547-87.

[27] Dedo HH, Fishman NH. Laryngeal release and sleeve resection for tracheal stenosis. Ann Otol Rhinol Laryngol. 1969; 78: 285-95.

[28] Rao PM, Noveline RA, Dobins JM. The spherical endotracheal tube cuff: A plain radiographic sign of tracheal injury. Emerg Radiol. 1996; 3: 87-90.

[29] Gonzalez RP, Falimirski M, Holevar MR, Turk B. Penetrating zone ll neck injury: Does dynamic computed tomographic scan contribute to the diagnostic sensitivity of physical examination for surgically significant injury? A prospective blinded study. J Trauma. 2003; 54: 61-5.

[30] Leopold DA: Laryngeal trauma, Arch Otolaryngol 1983; 109:106-109.

[31] Darlong LM, Shunyu NB, Das R, Malli KS. Cut throat zone ll injury and advantage of a feeding jejunostomy. J Emerg Trauma Shock. 2009; 2: 213-5.

[32] Litwack TR. Assessments of dangerousness: Legal research and clinical developments. Administration and-Policy-in-Mental-Health. 1994; 21: 361-377.

[33] Douglas K, Kropp P. A prevention-based paradigm for violence risk assessment: Clinical research application. Criminal Justice and Behaviour. 2002; 29: 617-658.

[34] Hart S. The role of psychopathy in assessing risk for violence: conceptual and methodological issues. Legal and Criminological Psychology. 1998; 3: 121-137.

[35] Ezeanolue BC.Management of the upper airway in severe cut throat injuries. African Journal of medicine and medical sciences 2001;30:233-5.18.

[36] Sett S, Isser DK. Laryngotracheal stenosis and pharyngocutaneous fistula in cut throat injuries: how we manage them. Indian J Otolaryngol Head Neck Surg. 2000; 52(3): 315-318.

[37] Mandour M, Remacle M, Van de heyning P, Elwany S, Tantawy A, Gaafar A. Chronic subglottic and tracheal stenosis: endoscopic management versus surgical reconstruction. Eur Arch Otorhinolaryngol. 2003; 260(7): 374-380.

Part 3

Conclusion – An Attempt at Integrating Understanding, Predicting, and Controlling

9

Selfhood: A Theory-Derived Relational Model for Mental Illness and Its Applications

Luciano L'Abate[1] and Mario Cusinato[2]
[1]Georgia State University
[2]University of Padova
[1]USA
[2]Italy

1. Introduction

The purpose of this chapter is to introduce a theory-derived relational model for Mental Illness and its applications in self-help, health-promotion, sickness prevention, and psychotherapy. Consequently, most of this chapter will be concerned with explaining and expanding on; (1) the basic theoretical derivation of this model, (2) its relational qualities and (3) views of mental health and mental illness, (4) research to validate its construct, convergent, and predictive validities; and (5) its clinical and preventive applications in mental health.

2. Theoretical origins of the Selfhood Model[11]

Selfhood Model[11] is one of the most important models in Relational Competence Theory (RCT). It is also one of the most validated models of RCT, even though all the models of RCT are just as important but perhaps not as important and as validated as Selfhood, as summarized in Figure 1. Furthermore, not all models lead to direct clinical, promotional, preventive, and psychotherapeutic applications as the model Selfhood. To fully explain this Model[11] it will not be necessary to spend as much space and time on the whole RCT. There are plenty of sources where this theory has been explained in greater detail (Cusinato & L'Abate, 2012; L'Abate, 2005; 2008a; 2009c; L'Abate & Cusinato, 2007; L'Abate, Cusinato, Maino, Colesso, & Scilletta, 2010).

It is important to underscore that the 16 model of RCT were created to encompass as many qualities as possible of relational competence relevant to both intimate and non-intimate relationships. The overall scheme is a hierarchical pyramidal flowchart or organizational chart because it needs to differentiate among meta-theoretical (Models[1-3]) from theoretical ([Model4-6]) assumptions as well as between developmentally normative (Models[7-12]) from non-normative Models[13-15]. Summary Model[16] about Negotiation includes both normative and non-normative charac-teristics that are present in all models ([1-15]) of RCT.

The historical origins of RCT in general and of the Selfhood Model[11] in particular go back to half a century ago, when behaviorism, psychoanalysis, and eventually humanism were in full force. Less known and less popular was systems theory and information processing formulations. The latter were very influential in starting to think about the family as the major system in existence. Influenced by the discipline of family sociology, that existence raised the question about why in psychology we did not have a specialty in "family psychology". Furthermore, why was there no theory to trying to understand behavior and relationships within the family system, except for empirically untestable psychoanalytic formulations?

At the beginning, influenced by the individual, intrapsychic paradigm, understanding and helping the individual in the family was the principal focus of the theory. From there, various revisions of the theory focused on popular terms, such as "Self", "Personality," and eventually "Family". However, even that latter term was not satisfactory because in USA only 25% of all domiciles are composed by the traditional, sociological notion of the intact marital couples and two children of opposite gender. The other 75% include various combinations and permutation of people living under the same roof linked by emotional, ethnic, financial, and practical ties.

Since the notion of family-qua-family was no longer tenable, the notion of "intimate" relationships was introduced as a substitute for the notion of "family". Intimate, communal relationships are characterized by close, committed, interdependent, and durable bonds. Non-intimate, agentic relationships are characterized by inadequacy and lack of closeness, commitment, interdependence, and duration. Furthermore, most psychological models about personality, marriage, and the family have produced a plethora of highly validated measures that are, however, specific only to either personalities, or couples, or families. Measures to evaluate individuals in a non-relational *vacuum* produced a veritable theoretical and empirical Tower of Babel in personality science. This Tower of Babel essentially considered personality in a relational vacuum, without any intimate or non-intimate relationships while marriages and families were viewed without personalities. There were essentially three different theoretical and empirical tracks without any connection among them. We needed a theory of human relationships that would go above and beyond personalities, couples, and families, a very ambitious but exciting undertaking that has been going on for the last half century.

Consequently, collaborators at the University of Padova, lead by the co-author of this chapter, Mario Cusinato and his students (Cusinato & L'Abate, 2012; L'Abate et al., 2010) agreed that we were interested in expanding and evaluating the validity a theory about human, relational competence that could and should be empirically evaluated and possibly validated. Eventually (L'Abate & Cusinato, 2007), we realized that in order to make sense of all the models that encompassed the undeniable complexity of RCT, we had to fall back and resort on Max Weber's century-old notion of hierarchy, as present in most charitable, educational, industrial, military, and religious organizations. Hence, we arrived at the hierarchy presented in Figure 1 below.

2.1 Requirements for RCT

These four requirements are necessary to understand the nature of RCT as: (1) *verifiable* model by model, like in any human organization, each model has to be accountable and has to be verified from the top down; (2) *applicable* to individuals, couples, and families as well as functional and dysfunctional conditions and relationships in different Settings (Model[3]); (3) *redundant* in linking models together to describe and explain one particular construct, all models are interrelated to support each other by expanding the meaning of a construct from the different viewpoints represented by each model; and (4) *fruitful* in producing research and applications to validate or invalidate its models, a requirement that implies also *longevity*.

The requirement of redundancy eventually will be useful to understand the inevitable and necessary overlap among dimensions of functionality-dysfunctionality, as shown at the conclusion of this chapter. Since this requirement is relatively new in psychological theory-construction, it might be relevant to expand on its meaning and function within a hierarchical, pyramidal theoretical framework. Redundancy, within the context of RCT, means that human relationships are too complex to be described, explained, or even understood by one single, solitary model. Those relationships can and should be evaluated, described, and perhaps even explained and eventually understood, from multiple but overlapping viewpoints or models. Each model, in and of itself, represents one different way to look at the same construct in relation with different viewpoints.

For instance, Model[4], deals with the ability to love, a multidimensional construct, described first according to a dimension of distance: who and what we approach or avoid, how often and for how long we approach someone or something we love or like and avoid someone or something we do not like. Second, an overlapping construct of love (Figure 1) is also found in Model[7], using a different set of dimensions in the Triangle of Life. This Triangle was derived from resource exchange theory (Foa, Converse, Tornblom, & Foa, 1993) composed of: (1) emotional and instrumental Being or Presence that includes Importance or Status (Model[11]) and Love or Intimacy (Model[15]): (2) Doing or Performance, composed of Information and Services; and (3) Having or Production, composed of Goods or Possessions and Money. In this model, Love is defined by Being Present and available reciprocally to those we love and who love us emotionally and instrumentally. Third, additionally, different meanings of love are visible in the Selfhood Model[11] described in this chapter, on how Importance is bestowed on self and intimates. Fourth, another meaning of love is found in Model[12] about Priorities: what kind of Priorities determine our behavior toward intimates and non-intimates? Fifth, another meaning is found in the Intimacy Model[15], defined as the sharing of joys and hurts and fears of being hurt. This sharing usually occurs at home and intimate relationships found there, not at work, in the office, or in bars or gyms.

The same kind of redundant analysis could be performed with Model[5] about the ability to control self is described by a dimension of speed, how fast or how slow we respond in approaching or avoiding people, responsibilities, or tasks. This Model[5] can be seen from the viewpoint of Model[7], according to whoever controls Doing and Having has the power to control others, as seen in most despots around the world. Control of self is also relevant to Model[16] about negotiation. One cannot negotiate adequately with others if one is not in full control of oneself.

2.2 Requirements for models of RCT

In addition to being verifiable and verified and being defined by the same requirements for RCT in general, RCT models can vary along a dimension of functionality/dysfunctionality, developmentally and normatively. Some models, such as Models[4, 5, 6, 7, 8, 9, 10, & 11] are definitely linked to Axis I and II of the DSM-IV, while Models[13, 14, & 15] in and of themselves unrelated to the DSM-IV evaluate and are linked directly to dysfunctional relationships and roles.

Furthermore, some models have been supported by *independent* evidence (face validity), such as secondary references completely unrelated to RCT but with sufficient similarity to RCT models to warrant their presume or suggestive validity (L'Abate, 2009a). Some models are supported by *indirect* evidence about the validity of the model. This would be the case,

Requirements					
Verifiability	Applicability		Redundancy	Fruitfulness	
Meta-theoretical Assumptions about Relationships					
	Width[1]		Depth[2]	Settings[3]	
Models	ERAAwC[1]		Levels of Interpretation[2]	Settings[3]	
	Emotionality		Description	Home	
	Rationality		Presentation	School/work	
	Activity		Phenotype	Transit	
	Awareness		Explanation	Transitory	
	Context		Genotype		
			Generational-developmental		
Theoretical Assumptions about Relationships					
Models	Ability to Love[4]	Ability to Control Self[5]	Both Abilities[6]	Contents[7]	
Dimensions	Distance	Control	Functionality	Modalities	
	Approach/Avoidance	Discharge/Delay	High/Middle/Low	Being/Doing/Having	
DSM-IV	Axis II, Cluster C	Axis II, Cluster B	GAF* (100 to 0)*	Sexual deviations / Driven Personalities	
Normative Models of the Theory					
Models	Self-differentiation[8]	Relational Styles[9]	Interactions[10]	Selfhood[11]	Priorities[12]
Dimensions	Likeness Continuum	AA/RR/CC	Functionality	Importance	Survival/Enjoyment
a.	Symbiosis/Alienation	Abusive/Apathetic	Divisive	No-self	Vertical: Self/intimates
b.	Sameness/Oppositeness	Reactive/Repetitive	Subtractive/Static	Selfless/Selfish	Horizontal: Settings
c.	Similarity/Differentness	Conductive/Creative	Additive/Multiplicative	Selfull	
DSM-IV	a. Axis I b. Axis II, Cluster B c. No diagnosis	a. Co-dependencies/addictions b. Conflict high c. Conflict low	a. Below 39 on GAF* b. 69 to 40 on GAF c. 100 to 70 on GAF * GAF= Global Assessment of Functioning		
Clinical Applications of the Theory					
Models	Distance Regulation[13]	Drama Triangle[14]	Intimacy[15]	Negotiation[16]	
Dimensions	Pursuer/Distancer/Regulator	Victim/Persecutor/Rescuer	Sharing Joys, Hurts, & Fears of Being hurt	Structure/Process (Ill, Skill, Will)	

Fig. 1. Summary of Relational Competence Theory

for instance, of Models [4, 5, & 6] where support is furnished from other sources or measures developed by researchers extraneous to RCT. Some models have produced specific, paper-and-pencil self-report measures that evaluate *directly* the psychometric robustness of each model (construct, concurrent, and predictive validities among others). This is especially the case for Models[1, 2, 3, 7, 11, 15, & 16]. Model[11] was evaluated also with a visual-verbal test for couples that needs further applications (Cusinato & L'Abate, 2005a, 2005b).

Some models have been expanded by revising original model-derived measures. For instance, the Relational Answers Questionnaire to evaluate Model[1] was revised and expanded from five (Emotionality, Rationality, Activity, Awareness, Context) to seven components of an information processing Model[1] (Cusinato, 2012). The importance of Emotionality as the basis of our humanity has lead to an entire series of studies about alexithymia, that is: the inability to experience feelings and therefore express them as emotions (Cusinato & L'Abate, 2012). Model[2], composed of two levels of : (1) description, with sublevels of (a) self-presentation/impression management façade and (b) behavior in intimate prolonged relationships; and (2) explanation with two sublevels (a) genotypical and (b) developmental/generational influences, can be evaluated with a revised Self-presentation scale (Cusinato, 2012).

Model[3] about various specific survival and enjoyment settings can be evaluated by a revised R-EcoMap that includes also evaluation of how the immediate relational contexts and intimates are perceived by participants (Colesso, 2012b). Model[8] about identity-differentiation has been originally evaluated in a face-to-face verbal administration that limited its being available to more than one individual at a time (Cusinato & Colesso, 2008). However, it has been expanded into a written format that allows mass administration at one time (Colesso, 2012a). Model[14] about the Deadly Drama Triangle (DDT) composed by the Victim, Perpetrator, and Rescuer has been expanded in a forthcoming volume that includes similar or related models, such as Parentification, when a child is assigned or assumes the parental role toward one's parents, the Parental Alienation Syndrome (PAS), when one parent demonizes the other, usually divorced parent with the children. Bullying, that has now reached epidemic proportions in the United States, and the Stockholm Syndrome, where one kidnapped individual assumes the role of the kidnappers (Hooper, L'Abate, Sweeney, Gianesini, & Jankoski, in press). Model[15] about intimacy already defined as the sharing of joys and hurts and fears of being hurt has been expanded into a full-fledged volume (L'Abate, 2011a).

Additionally, certain models are applied and validated when administered as Programmed Interactive Practice Exercises (PIPEs; L'Abate, 2004a, 2011) or workbooks require distance writing, as discussed below (L'Abate & Sweeney, 2011). Some PIPEs are completely independent from sources or models of RCT. Some PIPEs are related indirectly to models of RCT. Some PIPES are directly related to models of RCT, as discussed in greater detail below.

3. Relational qualities of Selfhood Model[11] and their connections with mental illness

This Selfhood Model[11] is based on the notion that a sense of importance is continuously exchanged between and among intimates and non-intimates. This exchange occurs through the bestowal of importance to Self and intimate Others. When this sense of importance is bestowed positively toward Self and Others, a relational propensity called *Selfulness* emerges, producing cooperative functionality in three major Settings (Model[3]), home (family), school/work, and surplus time. When a sense of importance is bestowed positively on Self more than negatively on Others, a relational propensity called *Selfishness* emerges leading to competitive derogation and impulsive devaluation of others based on envy, anger, acting out, aggression, and in its extremes, murder, as exemplified by personality disorders of Axis II Cluster B from the DSM-IV (Fisher & Cox, 2011; Madden && Bickel, 2010). When a sense of importance is bestowed negatively on Self and positively on Others, a relational propensity called *Selflessness* emerges, leading to sadness, depression, anxiety, and in its extreme suicide, as exemplified by personality disorders of Axis II Cluster C of the DSM-IV. When a sense of importance is bestowed negatively on both Self and Others, a relational propensity called *No-self* emerges, leading to various psychopathological conditions, as exemplified by Axis I and Axis II Cluster A disorders of the DSM-IV.

Possible gender differences were predicted from the very outset of RCT (L'Abate, 1994), with men being trained relatively more than women to behave selfishly and women being trained relatively more than men to behave selflessly. Equal gender ratios are predicted for Selfulness as well as for No-Self.

This Selfhood Model[11], as shown in Figure 2, integrates various degrees of functionality (Selfulness) and different degrees and types of dysfunctionalities, providing a relational, dimensional version of static, non-dimensional psychiatric categories of the DSM-IV.

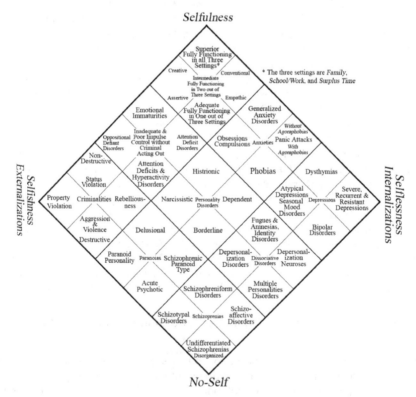

Fig. 2. Integration of Psychiatric Categories with Relational Dimensions and Expansion to Superior Functioning

4. Research to validate the Selfhood Model[11]

Most of the research to evaluate the psychometric validities of this model has been conducted with various versions of the Self-Other-Profile Chart (SOPC). The latest version is shown in Figure 3. Most of the research to validate this SOPC has been conducted at the University of Padova under the leadership of the second author (Cusinato & L'Abate, 2012; L'Abate et al., 2010, pp. 163-188).

The convergent and construct validities of this model were evaluated with the SOPC in 19 different studies, using instruments already validated in English, mostly in USA. Seven studies evaluated the construct validity of the SOPC. Five studies supported the hypothesis of possible gender differences, with men appearing more selfish than women. Fourteen studies evaluated also the convergent/divergent validity of the SOPC. Results from these studies tend to confirm the convergent, criterion, and construct validities of this instrument and, therefore, of the Model[11] underlying it. Current research (Cusinato & L'Abate, 2012) is validating a newer and more complete version of this instrument, as shown in Figure 3.

In previous studies (L'Abate, 1997), this instrument was found to correlate significantly with much lengthier self-concept tests, like the Tennessee Self-Concept. In a sample of 100 parents of elementary school children (Salvo, 1998): (a) Selflessness correlates ($r = .12$, $p < .05$) with Dismissing style on the Adult Attachment Questionnaire; (b) Selfish propensity correlates significantly with all four attachment styles: $r = -.19$, $p < .01$ with Secure, $r = .15$, $p < .05$ with Preoccupied, $r = .27$, $p < .01$ with Dismissing, and $r = .18$, $p < .01$ for Fearful; (c) No-self shows significant correlations with the four attachment styles: $r = -.23$, $p < .01$ with Secure, $r = .27$, $p < .001$ with Preoccupied, $r = .25$, $p < .001$ with Dismissing, and $r = .29$, $p < .001$ with Fearful; (d) Selfulness correlates negatively with Selflessness ($r = -.29$, $p < .001$) but not with the other two propensities. Selflessness correlated positively with Selfishness ($r = .12$, $p < .05$) and with No-self ($r = .29$, $p < .001$). Selfishness and No-self correlated with each other ($r = .39$, $p < .01$).

A previous version of the SOPC was administered also to a group of primarily female (81.5%) adults (n = 153) with a mean age of 23 (Self Profile has $\alpha = .82$ and Other Profile has $\alpha = .83$; in test-retest Self Profile reliability is $r = .62$, Other Profile reliability is $r = .64$). Correlations with the Beck Depression Inventory (BDI) and with the Center for Epidemiological Studies Depression Scale (CES-D) are significant: Self Profile correlates negatively with BDI ($r = -.57$, $p < .001$) and CES-D ($r = -.55$, $p < .001$); Others Profile correlates significantly and negatively with BDI ($r = -.57$, $p < .001$) and CES-D($r = -.49$, $p < .001$).

4.1 Validation of the Revised SOPC$_2$ (Cusinato, 2012)

The first SOPC$_2$ administration involved 376 participants living in North Italy, aged from 14 to 55 years ($M = 30.44$, $SD = 11.48$), 184 (48.8%) males and 193 (51.2%) female, with various levels of education, status, and profession: (a) education: 67 (17.7%) with primary school level, 31 (8.2%) with professional diploma, 163 (43.2%) with a high school diploma, 116 (30.7%) with an university degree; (b) status: 107 singles (28.4%), 112 (29.7%) engaged, 26 (6.9%) living together, 120 (31.8%) married, 8 (2.1%) divorced, 3 (.8%) remarried, 1 (.3%) widowed; (c) occupation: 40 (10.6%) managers or similar, 70 (18.6%) clerks or similar, 27 (7.2%) http://it.dicios.com/iten/lavoratore-in-proprioself-employed workers, 66 (17.5%) http://it.dicios.com/iten/operaio-specializzatocraftsmen, 14 (3.7) unemployed, 145 (38.5) students, 14 (3.7) home crafts.

First Part: The Self Profile (SOPC-2, february, 2011)

Here is a list of quality related to people in general. You are asked two things in succession (before step 1 and then step 2):

Step 1: In column A, mark Yes if you believe that the quality is applicable to some extent to people like you (considering sex, age, education and living conditions) and NO if it is not. Please evaluate one by one all qualities proposed.

Step 2: Apply yourself the qualities chosen with YES and answer the following question (please use the scale beside):

How much these qualities makes me feel important?

→ continue

	LIST OF PERSONAL QUALITIES	A	rating scale					LIST OF PERSONAL QUALITIES	A	rating scale			
			little	enough	a lot	very much				little	enough	a lot	very much
1	Body Care	YES NO	1	2	3	4	34	Inventiveness	YES NO	1	2	3	4
2	Intelligence	YES NO	1	2	3	4	35	Kindness	YES NO	1	2	3	4
3	Affection	YES NO	1	2	3	4	36	Capacity to Work Together	YES NO	1	2	3	4
4	Friendliness	YES NO	1	2	3	4	37	Spirituality	YES NO	1	2	3	4
5	Consistency	YES NO	1	2	3	4	38	Initiative	YES NO	1	2	3	4
6	Concreteness	YES NO	1	2	3	4	39	Love for Nature	YES NO	1	2	3	4
7	Aesthetic Taste	YES NO	1	2	3	4	40	Awareness of owns Limits	YES NO	1	2	3	4
8	Beware of the Consequences	YES NO	1	2	3	4	41	Physical Strength	YES NO	1	2	3	4
9	Sex-appeal	YES NO	1	2	3	4	42	Intuition	YES NO	1	2	3	4
10	Memory	YES NO	1	2	3	4	43	Joyfulness	YES NO	1	2	3	4
11	Kindness	YES NO	1	2	3	4	44	Ability to Give Consideration	YES NO	1	2	3	4
12	Expansiveness	YES NO	1	2	3	4	45	Religiosity	YES NO	1	2	3	4
13	Commitment	YES NO	1	2	3	4	46	Sense of Business	YES NO	1	2	3	4
14	Common Sense	YES NO	1	2	3	4	47	Love for Dance	YES NO	1	2	3	4
15	Love for the Art	YES NO	1	2	3	4	48	Attention to Situations	YES NO	1	2	3	4
16	Ability to Reflect on the Experiences	YES NO	1	2	3	4	49	Resistance to fatigue	YES NO	1	2	3	4
17	Good Looks	YES NO	1	2	3	4	50	Curiosity	YES NO	1	2	3	4
18	Creativity	YES NO	1	2	3	4	51	Intimacy	YES NO	1	2	3	4
19	Empathy	YES NO	1	2	3	4	52	Sense of Friendship	YES NO	1	2	3	4
20	Sense of humor	YES NO	1	2	3	4	53	Sense of Family	YES NO	1	2	3	4
21	Green Think	YES NO	1	2	3	4	54	Crafts	YES NO	1	2	3	4
22	Methodicalness	YES NO	1	2	3	4	55	Musical Ear	YES NO	1	2	3	4
23	Love for the Music	YES NO	1	2	3	4	56	Ability to Learn from the Experiences	YES NO	1	2	3	4
24	Consciousness of owns Abilities	YES NO	1	2	3	4	57	Healthy Care	YES NO	1	2	3	4
25	Qualities in Sport	YES NO	1	2	3	4	58	Interest in Science	YES NO	1	2	3	4
26	Problem Solving	YES NO	1	2	3	4	59	Sharing Capacity	YES NO	1	2	3	4
27	Warmth in Relationships	YES NO	1	2	3	4	60	Opening for Social Life	YES NO	1	2	3	4
28	Leadership	YES NO	1	2	3	4	61	Generosity	YES NO	1	2	3	4
29	Respect in Relationships	YES NO	1	2	3	4	62	Ability to Carry out	YES NO	1	2	3	4
30	Professionalism	YES NO	1	2	3	4	63	Taste for the Beautiful	YES NO	1	2	3	4
31	Love for Poetry	YES NO	1	2	3	4	64	Attention to how Others Are	YES NO	1	2	3	4
32	Knowledge of the Capabilities of Others	YES NO	1	2	3	4							
33	Care of Health	YES NO	1	2	3	4							

Second Part: The Other Profile (SOPC-2, february 2011)

Here is a list of persons possible partners of close, committed, and prolonged relationships. You are asked two things in succession (before step 1 and then step 2):

Step 1: In A column, mark Yes if you believe that the relationship with this person is possible for one like you .(considering sex, age, education and living conditions) and NO if it is not. Please evaluate one by one all people proposed.

Step 2: Please consider the persons signed with Yes and answer the following question (please use the scale beside):

How much these persons make me feel important?

→ continue

	LIST OF PERSONS IN CLOSE, COMMITTED, AND PROLONGED RELATIONSHIPS	A	rating scale little / enough / a lot / very much					LIST OF PERSONS IN CLOSE, COMMITTED, AND PROLONGED RELATIONSHIPS	A	rating scale little / enough / a lot / very much			
1	Father	YES NO	1	2	3	4	34	Teammate	YES NO	1	2	3	4
2	Mother	YES NO	1	2	3	4	35	Car Engineering	YES NO	1	2	3	4
3	Grandfather	YES NO	1	2	3	4	36	Nurse	YES NO	1	2	3	4
4	Grandmother	YES NO	1	2	3	4	37	Family Doctor	YES NO	1	2	3	4
5	Husband	YES NO	1	2	3	4	38	Doctor in Attendance	YES NO	1	2	3	4
6	Wife	YES NO	1	2	3	4	39	Dentist	YES NO	1	2	3	4
7	Son	YES NO	1	2	3	4	40	Medical Specialist	YES NO	1	2	3	4
8	Daughter	YES NO	1	2	3	4	41	Accountant	YES NO	1	2	3	4
9	Brother	YES NO	1	2	3	4	42	Banking Consultant	YES NO	1	2	3	4
10	Sister	YES NO	1	2	3	4	43	Pastor	YES NO	1	2	3	4
11	Nephew	YES NO	1	2	3	4	44	Curate	YES NO	1	2	3	4
12	Uncle	YES NO	1	2	3	4	45	Association President	YES NO	1	2	3	4
13	Aunt	YES NO	1	2	3	4	46	Member of the Association	YES NO	1	2	3	4
14	Cousin (male)	YES NO	1	2	3	4	47	Neighbor	YES NO	1	2	3	4
15	Cousin (female)	YES NO	1	2	3	4	48	Head of Condominium	YES NO	1	2	3	4
16	Father-in-law	YES NO	1	2	3	4	49	Servant	YES NO	1	2	3	4
17	Mother-in-law	YES NO	1	2	3	4	50	Barber / Hairdresser	YES NO	1	2	3	4
18	Son-in-low	YES NO	1	2	3	4	51	Baby-sitter	YES NO	1	2	3	4
19	Sister-in-low	YES NO	1	2	3	4	52	Greengrocer	YES NO	1	2	3	4
20	Boy/Girlfriend	YES NO	1	2	3	4	53	Social Worker	YES NO	1	2	3	4
21	Childhood friend	YES NO	1	2	3	4	54	Teacher	YES NO	1	2	3	4
22	Friend of family	YES NO	1	2	3	4	55	Clerk of the Usual Shop	YES NO	1	2	3	4
23	Personal friend	YES NO	1	2	3	4	56	Barman/maid of the Usual Bar	YES NO	1	2	3	4
24	Partner	YES NO	1	2	3	4	57	Counselor	YES NO	1	2	3	4
25	School Colleague	YES NO	1	2	3	4	58	Psychologist	YES NO	1	2	3	4
26	Professor	YES NO	1	2	3	4	59	Maid of the usual restaurant	YES NO	1	2	3	4
27	Work Colleague	YES NO	1	2	3	4	60	Another person to mention*:	YES NO	1	2	3	4
28	Employer	YES NO	1	2	3	4	61	Another person to mention*:	YES NO	1	2	3	4
29	Superior	YES NO	1	2	3	4	62	Another person to mention*:	YES NO	1	2	3	4
30	Employee of the office usually attended	YES NO	1	2	3	4	63	Another person to mention*:	YES NO	1	2	3	4
31	Inferior	YES NO	1	2	3	4	64	Another person to mention*:	YES NO	1	2	3	4
32	Catechist	YES NO	1	2	3	4							
33	Coacher	YES NO	1	2	3	4							

continue →

* if you have to mention another brother, uncle, cousin, friend, colleague ... in addition to the already marked.

Self Profile: Quality Connection to the Areas

	AREAS					AREAS		
A	Physical Qualities	1	Body Care		E	Moral Qualities	5	Consistency
		9	Sex-appeal				13	Commitment
		17	Good Looks				21	Green Think
		25	Qualities in Sport				29	Respect in Relationships
		33	Care of Health				37	Spirituality
		41	Physical Strength				45	Religiosity
		49	Resistance to fatigue				53	Sense for family
		57	Healthy Care				61	Generosity
B	Cognitive Qualities	2	Intelligence		F	Performance Qualities	6	Concreteness
		10	Memory				14	Common Sense
		18	Creativity				22	Methodicalness
		26	Problem Solution				30	Professionalism
		34	Inventiveness				38	Initiative
		42	Intuition				46	Sense of Business
		50	Curiosity				54	Crafts
		58	Interest in Science				62	Ability to Carry out
C	Affective Qualities	3	Affection		G	Aesthetic Qualities	7	Aesthetic Taste
		11	Kindness				15	Love for the Art
		19	Empathy				23	Love for the Music
		27	Warmth in Relationships				31	Love for Poetry
		35	Kindness				39	Love for Nature
		43	Joyfulness				47	Love for Dance
		51	Intimacy				55	Musical Ear
		59	Sharing Capacity				63	Taste for the Beautiful
D	Social Qualities	4	Friendliness		H	Reflective Qualities	8	Beware of the Consequences
		12	Expansiveness				16	Ability to Reflect on the Experiences
		20	Sense of humor				24	Consciousness of owns Abilities
		28	Leadership				32	Knowledge of the Capabilities of Others
		36	Capacity to Work Together				40	Awareness of owns Limits
		44	Ability to Give Consideration				48	Attention to Situations
		52	Sense of Friendship				56	Ability to Learn from the Experiences
		60	Opening for Social Life				64	Attention to how Others Are

Other Profile: People Connection to the 4 Settings (first tentative)

	Home		Work		Survival		Enjoyment
1	Father	25	School Colleague	35	Car Engineering	21	Childhood friend
2	Mother	26	Professor	36	Nurse	22	Friend of family
3	Grandfather	27	Work Colleague	37	Family Doctor	23	Personal friend
4	Grandmother	28	Employer	38	Doctor in Attendance	32	Catechist
5	Husband	29	Superior	39	Dentist	33	Coacher
6	Wife	30	Employee of the office usually attended	40	Medical Specialist	43	Pastor
7	Son	31	Inferior	41	Accountant	44	Curate
8	Daughter	34	Teammate	42	Banking Consultant	45	Association President
9	Brother	54	Teacher	48	Head of Condominium	46	Member of the Association
10	Sister			49	Servant ??	47	Neighbor ??
11	Nephew			50	Barber / Hairdresser		
12	Uncle			51	Baby-sitter	51	Baby-sitter
13	Aunt			52	Greengrocer		
14	Cousin (male)			53	Social Worker		
15	Cousin (female)			55	Clerk of the Usual Shop	55	Clerk of the Usual Shop
16	Father-in-law			56	Barman/maid of the Usual Bar	56	Barman/maid of the Usual Bar
17	Mother-in-law			57	Counselor	57	Counselor
18	Son-in-low			58	Psychologist		
19	Sister-in-low			59	Maid of the usual restaurant	59	Maid of the usual restaurant
24	Partner						

Fig. 3.

The questionnaire was administered during the months of April 2011. The correct procedure was observed with appropriate letters of invitation, informed consent, instructions to perform the answer-sheets and collect the fulfilled questionnaires. The collected data were processed in May 2011 with the check of sample distribution, the reliability of the scales, the correlation analyses between profiles and areas, the analysis of variance with independent variables, the translation of the two profiles Self on Other in the propensities selfhood.

4.2 Results of the study

After determining the existence of a normal distribution in the data (Self Profile: asym. -. 08, Curt. .7; Other Profile: asym. -.27, Curt. .26), the analysis focused on the reliability of the profiles, the areas of personal qualities, and the people subdivided by settings. The results (Table 1) show coherent and consistent trends. The correlations between the profiles and the quality areas meet the expectations driving the construction of the instrument (Table 2 and Table 3). The correlation between the two profiles is positive and statistically significant (r = .41**). Therefore, the new version of SOPC seems to be reliable, even though further tests of reliability and validity (concurrent and differentiating in particular) will be performed in the future. The time spent to compile the two profiles seems to be acceptable: mean = 17 min. (range 8-30 min).

	M	SD	α
Self Profile	**202.10**	**32.94**	**.92**
Physical qualities	22.65	5.40	.64
Cognitive qualities	26.31	5.34	.68
Affettive qualities	27.85	5.97	.79
Social qualities	27.86	5.02	.68
Moral qualities	26.22	5.96	.76
Performance qualities	24.51	6.35	.70
Esthetic qualities	20.21	6.12	.73
Riflexive qualities	26.51	6.28	.77
Other Profile	**133.73**	**29.55**	**.85**
People related to home	50.16	14.08	.85
People related to work	17.99	5.80	.73
People related to survival settings	31.37	10.75	.88
People related to enjoyment settings	26.09	6.54	.71

Table 1. Means, Standard Deviation, and Internal Consistency of Profiles and Areas/Settings

	Phys.	Cogn.	Affet.	Soc.	Moral	Perf.	Esth.	Riflex.
Self Profile	.59**	.78**	.77**	.69**	.76**	.72**	.61**	.73**
Other Profile	.21**	.30**	.31**	.28**	.30**	.25**	.32**	.31**

** = p .01

Table 2. Correlations between Profiles and Quality Areas

	Home	Work	Surv.S.	Enj.S.
Self Profile	.29**	.33**	.39**	.30**
Other Profile	.82**	.75**	.81**	.73**

** = p .01

Table 3. Correlations between Profiles and Quality Areas

4.3 The step from propensity to selfhood propensities

A particularly interesting aspect of these results deserves to be proposed for applications in training and clinical practices. On a formal level, the derivation of selfhood propensities of the two profiles has been chosen according to the criteria shown in Figure 4. At the operational level, percentiles 16th and 84th are identified (in theory correspondent to one SD less and more to mean in the standardized Gauss curve) as a cut-off point into three parts. This procedure can obtain 9 types of which 4 correspond to the earlier model of selfhood propensities and the others are intermediate positions, except for the central that could be considered as indecision.

	-	**Self Profile**	+
+	selfless	selfless-selfull	selfull
Other Profile	nearly selfless	middle selfhood	selfull-selfish
-	no-self	nearly selfish	selfish

Fig. 4. Derivation of selfhood propensities from the two Profiles

The intersection of the three levels of Self and Other Profiles with the significance calculated using log-linear analyses gave the results shown by Table 4.

selfless	selfless-selfull	selfull
0	31 (8.38%)	22 (5.95%)
-3.02**	-0.25	-0.13
nearly selfless	middle selfhood	selfull-selfish
50 (13.51%)	173 (46.76%)	31 (8.38%)
4.56**	10.98**	3.14**
no-self	nearly selfish	selfish
16 (4.32%)	46 (12.43)	1 (.27%)
0.36	5.22**	-2.92**

** p = .01

Table 4. Derivation of extreme and intermediate propensities in Selfhood

As a consistent result with this procedure, data are distributed mainly in the intermediate range; the two propensities selfless and selfish appear somewhat extreme because 47% of the processed data is not oriented towards specific propensities. The orientation towards selfish, selfless, and selfull is significantly present.

The new version of the Self-Other-Profile Chart seems at first blush more complex and more complicated than the original version. On the other hand, it seems to cover many more relevant areas of Selfhood, including also relationships to Model2, where a distinction was made between servival and enjoyment settings. The acceptable psychometric properties of this revision allow an expansion of the original Model[11] that seems closer to the real-life realities of everyday living.

5. Clinical and preventive applications of the Selfhood Model[11] in mental health

Clinical and preventive applications of the Selfhood Model[11] are based on programmed distance writing occurring through computers and the Internet (L'Abate, 2011c, 2012; L'Abate & Sweeney, 2011) through replicable workbooks or programmed or interactive practice exercises (PIPEs). These exercises can be administered either as substitutes for or in addition to face-to-face talk in the promotion of mental and physical health, prevention of mental illness, or treatment and rehabilitation of mental illness. These PIPEs have been developed from a variety of sources, including research on anxiety, depression, Clusters B and C conditions, and from most dysfunctional conditions available in Axis I of the Diagnostic and Statistical Manual for Mental Illness-IV, including also factor analyses, single- and multiple score tests, such as the Beck Depression Inventory, and the Minnesota Multiphasic Personality Inventory, among many other tests and questionnaire

The transformation from inert paper-and-pencil self-report instruments and measures into active and interactive workbooks (L'Abate, 2011c) is obtained by asking participants to define items in any list of behaviors or symptoms, using the dictionary (L'Abate, 2007) if necessary, and then giving two examples from the definition, a nomothetic step. After completing this first step, participants are asked to rank-order items according to their importance to them, an idiographic step. This rank-order is used to administer following PIPEs according to a standard format that includes specific questions about the developmental origins, frequency, intensity, duration, rate and personal and relational outcomes of that particular behavior.

This transformation allows to change most evaluative instruments into active and interactive workbooks, thus linking and matching evaluation with intervention in ways that would be difficult if not impossible to achieve as long as face-to-face talk based on personal contact is the norm for most clinical, promotional, preventive, rehabilitative, and therapeutic practices. This transformation was specifically applied to a previous and simpler version of the SOPC thus linking directly a model of RCT to evaluation and to intervention (L'Abate, 2011c). This latest version could be transformed by any mental health professional into a interactive practice exercise using the guidelines given in the previous paragraph.

The usefulness of these PIPEs has been evaluated in various studies (L'Abate, 2004b) and in a meta-analysis by Smyth and L'Abate (2001), where the effect-size of these workbooks was found to be .44. In addition to clinical experience and case studies included in L'Abate (2011c), this effect size indicates that it is possible to change behavior for the better through programmed distance writing without ever seeing or talking with a participant face-to-face, provided that the interactive practice exercises match the condition in need of improvement (L'Abate, 2008b, 2008c).

6. Relationship of PIPEs to the Selfhood Model[11]

The relationship between PIPEs and Selfhood Model[11] is shown in Figure 5. This figure integrates most normative and non-normative PIPEs, regardless of theoretical orientation, gender, and educational level.

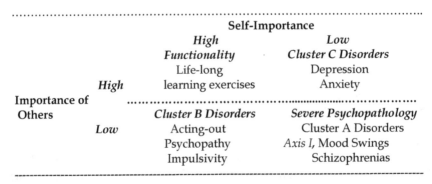

Fig. 5. Relationships among Selfhood Relational Propensities, Functionality, Psychopathology (DSM-IV), and Sample Interactive Practice Excises (L'Abate, 2011c)

7. Conclusion

If just one Selfhood Model[11] from RCT can accomplish this much, one cannot help wondering what the other 15 models of RCT can be accomplish. As mentioned repeatedly during the course of this chapter, practically every model of RCT attempts to cover functional and dysfunctional conditions. For instance, Model[8], about identity differentiation covers functional and dysfunctional conditions derived directly from the developmental notion of "same-different" (Figure 1). Using the requirement of redundancy introduced at the beginning of this chapter, the six ranges of the Likeness continuum in Model[8] (symbiosis, sameness, similarity/differentness, oppositeness, and alienation), were expanded into three relational Styles in Model[9], Conductive-Creative (CC), Reactive-Repetitive (RR), and Abusive-Apathetic (AA), and in six types of interactions in an arithmetical Model[10]: multiplicative, additive, static positive, static negative, subtractive, and divisive.

An interesting feature of Model[10] relates to the ratio of these six interactions with the presence of hurt feelings and intimacy defined earlier in this chapter (Cusinato & L'Abate, 2012; L'Abate, 2011a; L'Abate et al., 2010). These ratios are relevant to both mental health and mental illness. For instance, in multiplicative interactions the ratio of joys to hurts would be 6 to 1, in additive interactions the ratio would be 5 to 2, in static positive interactions the ratio would be 4 to 3, in static negative 3 to 4, in subtractive 2 to 5, and in divisive interactions 1 or 0 to 6. This model, therefore, views mental illness as the outcome of hurts offsetting joys and mental health as the outcome of joys offsetting hurts. These models overlap redundantly with the Selfhood Model[11] in producing a classification of relationships, as shown in Figure 6.

Figure 6 shows how human relationships can be classified according to relational (rather than intrapsychic and non-relational), dimensions that cover and encompass the whole gamut of mental health and mental illness. This classification of relationships among human

		Model[7]: Continuum of Likeness		
Symbiosis	Sameness	Similarity/Differentness	Oppositeness	Alienation

		Model[8]: Styles in Intimate Relationships		
Abusive Apathetic	Reactive Repetitive	Conductive Creative	Reactive Repetitive	Abusive Apathetic

		Model[9]: Interactions		
Divisive/ Subtractive	Static/ Positive	Multiplicative/ Additive	Static/ Negative	Divisive/ Subtractive

		Model[10]: Selfhood		
No-self	Selfish/Selfless	Selfful	Selfish/Selfless	No-self

		Psychiatric Categories (DSM-IV)		
Axis I & Axis II/ Cluster A	*Axis II Clusters B & C*	*No diagnoses*	*Axis II Clusters B & C*	*Axis I & Axis II/ Cluster A*

*Adapted from L'Abate et al., (2010).

Fig. 6. Relationships among four Models of Identity Differentiation[7], Styles[8], Interactions[9], and Selfhood[10]*

beings can be applied to individuals separate from couples, or to couples separate from families. We do not need separate and different tests or theories to understand separately individuals, couples, or families because in one way or anther these relationships can be understood in terms of these and other dimensions of the RCT models. This classification, of course, implies learning a completely new vocabulary that is based on models evaluated empirically in many different ways and found valid and reliable in observing and understanding mental health and mental illness on various dynamic continua or dimensions rather static categories.

8. References

Aboujaoude, E., & Koran, L. M. (2010). *Impulse control disorders.* New York: Cambridge University Press.

Author (1994). *Diagnostic Statistical Manual for Mental Disorders-IV.* Washington, DC: American Psychiatric Association Press.

Baumeister, R. F., &Vohs, K. D. (Eds.). (2004). *Handbook of self-regulation: Research, theory, and applications.* New York: Guilford.

Berreby, D. (2008). *US & THEM: The science of identity.* Chicago, IL: University of Chicago Press.

Beutler, L. E., &Malik, M. L. (Eds.). (2002*). Rethinking the DSM-IV: A psychological perspective.* Washington, DC: American Psychological Association.

Broffenbrenner, U. (1989). Toward an experimental ecology of human behavior. *American Psychologist, 32,* 513-531.

Cacioppo, J. T., & Gardner, W. L. (1999). Emotion. *Annual Review of Psychology, 50,* 191-214.

Canary, D. J., Emmers-Sommer, T. M., & Faulkner, D. (1997). *Sex and gender differences in personal relationships.* New York: Guilford.

Clark, M. S., & Mills, J. (1979). Interpersonal attraction in exchange and communal relationships. *Journal of Personality and Social Psychology, 37,* 12-24.

Clark, M. S., Pataki, S. P., & Carver, V. H. (1996). Some thoughts and findings on self-presentation of emotions in relationships. In G. J. O. Fletcher & J. Fitness (Eds.), *Knowledge structures in close relationships: A social psychological appraisal* (pp. 247-324). New York: Guilford.

Cocking, R. R., &Renninger, K. A. (Eds.). (1993). *The development and meaning of psychological distance.*Hillsdate, NJ: Erlbaum.

Cole, T., &Teboul, JC. B. (2004). Non-zero-sum collaboration, reciprocity, and the preference for similarity. *Personal Relationships, 11,* 135-160.

Colesso, W. (2012a). Continuum of likeness scales: New proposal for evaluating self-identity differentiation. In M. Cusinato & L'Abate (Eds.), *Advances in relational competence theory: With special attention to alexithymia* (pp. 00-00). New York; Nova Science Publishers.

Colesso, W. (2012b). Updating the R-C-EcoMap. In M. Cusinato & L'Abate (Eds.), *Advances in relational competence theory: With special attention to alexithymia* (pp. 00-00). New York; Nova Science Publishers.

Csikszentmihaly, M. (2004). Materialism and the evolution of consciousness. In T. Kasser& A. D. Kanner (Eds.), *Psychology and consumer culture: The struggle for a good life in a materialistic world* (pp. 91-106). Washington, DC: American Psychological Association.

Cunningham, M. R., Shamblen, S. R., Barbee, A. P., & Ault, L. K. (2005). Social allergies in romantic relationships: Behavioral repetition, emotional sensitization, and dissatisfaction in dating couples. *Personal Relationships, 12,* 273-295.

Cusinato, M. (2012a). A new version of the Self-Other-Profile-Chart. . In M. Cusinato & L'Abate (Eds.), *Advances in relational competence theory: With special attention to alexithymia* (pp. 00-00). New York; Nova Science Publishers.

Cusinato, M. (2012b). Self-presentation strategies: A new version of the self-presentation scale. In M. Cusinato & L'Abate (Eds.), *Advances in relational competence theory: With special attention to alexithymia* (pp. 00-00). New York; Nova Science Publishers.

Cusinato, M., & Colesso, W. (2008). Validation of the continuum of likeness in intimate relationships. In L. L'Abate (Ed.), *Toward a science of clinical psychology: Laboratory evaluations and interventions* (pp. 335-352). Hauppauge, NY: Nova Science Publishers.

Cusinato, M., & L'Abate, L. (2005a).The Dyadic Relationships Test: Creation and validation of a model-derived, visual-verbal instrument to evaluate couple relationships. Part I of II. *American Journal of Family Therapy, 33,* 195-206.

Cusinato, M., & L'Abate, L. (2005b). The Dyadic Relationships Test: Creation and validation of a model-derived, visual-verbal instrument to evaluate couple relationships. Part II. *American Journal of Family Therapy, 33,* 379-394.

Cusinato, M., & L'Abate, L. (Eds.). (2012). *Advances in relational competence theory: With special attention to alexithymia.* New York: Nova Science Publishers.

Davis, R., &Millon, T. (1995). On the importance of theory to a taxonomy of personality disorders. In J. W. Livesley (Ed.), *The DSM-IV personality disorders* (pp. 377-396). New York: Guilford.

Deal, J. E., Halverson, C. F. Jr., &Wampler, K. S. (1999). Parental similarity on child-rearing orientations: Effects of stereotype similarity. *Journal of Social and Personal Relationships, 16,* 87-102.

De Giacomo, P., L'Abate, L., Pennebaker, J. M., & D. M. Rumbaugh, D. M. (2010). From A to D: Ampli-fications and applications of Pennebaker'sanalogic to digital model in health promotion, prevention, and psychotherapy. *Clinical Psychology & Psychotherapy, 17,* 355-362.

Esterling, B. A., L'Abate, L., Murray, E., & Pennebaker, J. M. (1999). Empirical foundations for writing in prevention and psychotherapy: Mental and physical outcomes. *Clinical Psychology Review, 19,* 79-96.

Feeney, J. A. (1999). Issues of closeness and distance in dating relationships: Effects of sex and attachment style. *Journal of Social and Personal Relationships, 16,* 571-590.

Fincham, F. D., & Beach, S. R. H. (2002a). Forgiveness in marriage: Implications for psychological aggression and constructive communication. *Personal Relationships, 9,* 239-251.

Fisher, M., & Cox, A. (2011). Four strategies used during intrasexual competition for mates. *Personal Relationships, 18,* 20-38.

Flett, G. L., & Hewitt, P. L. (Eds.). (2002). *Perfectionism: Theory, research, and treatment.* Washington, DC: American Psychological Association.

Foa, U. G., Converse, J. Jr., Tornblom, K. J., &. Foa, E. B. (Eds.). (1993). *Resource exchange theory: Explorations and applications.* San Diego, CA: Academic Press.

Gable, S. L., Reis, S. T., & Elliot, A. J. (2000). Behavioral activation and inhibition in everyday life. *Journal of Personality and Social Psychology, 78,* 1135-1149.

Grisham, J. R., & Barlow, D. H. (2005). Compulsive hoarding: Current research and theory. *Journal of Psychopathology and Behavioral Assessment, 27,* 45-52.

Guinote, A., &Veschio, T. K. (Eds.). (2010). *The social psychology of power.* New York: Guildford.

Harter, S., Waters, P. I., Pettitt, L. M.,Whitesell, J. K., & Jordan, J. (1997). Autonomy and connectedness as dimensions of relationship styles in men and women. *Journal of Social and Personal Relationships, 14,* 147-164.

Harwood, T. M., & L'Abate, L. (2010). *Self-help in mental health: A critical evaluation.* New York: Springer-Science.

Hess, J. A., Fannin, A. D., &Pollom, L. H. (2007). Creating closeness: Discerning and measuring strategies for fostering closer relationships. *Personal Relationships, 14,* 24-44.

Hooper, L., L'Abate, L., Sweeney, L. G., Gianesini, G., & Jankoski, P. (in press). *Models of psychopathology: Generational and relational processes.* New York: Springer-Science.

Horowitz, L. M. (2004). *Interpersonal foundations of psychopathology.* Washington, DC: American Psychological Association.

Impett, E. A., Peplau, L. A., & Gable, S. L. (2005). Approach and avoidance sexual motives: Implications for personal and interpersonal well-being. *Personal Relationships, 12,* 465-482.

Jung Suh, E., Moskowitz, D. S., Fournier, M. A., & Zuroff, D. C. (2004). Gender and relationships: Influences on agentic and communal behaviors. *Personal Relationships, 11,* 41-59.

Kazantzis, N., Deane, F. P., Ronan, K. R., & L'Abate, L. (Eds.). (2005). *Using homework assignments in cognitive behavior therapy.* New York: Rutledge.

Kazantzis, N., & L'Abate, L. (Eds.). (2007). *Handbook of homework assignments in psychotherapy: Theory, research, and prevention.* New York: Springer-Science.

Kochalka, J., & L'Abate, L. (1997). Linking evaluation with structured enrichment: The Family Profile Form. *American Journal of Family Therapy, 25,* 361-374.

Krueger, R. F., & Tackett, J. L. (Eds.). (2006). *Personality and psychopathology.* New York: Guilford.

L'Abate, L. (1997b). *The self in the family: A classification of personality, criminality, and psychopathology.* New York: Wiley.

L'Abate, L. (1999). Taking the bull by the horns: Beyond talk in psychological interventions. *The Family Journal: Counseling and Therapy for Couples and Families,7,* 206-220.

L'Abate, L. (2004a). *A guide to self-help workbooks for clinicians and researchers.* Binghamton, NY: Haworth.

L'Abate, L. (Ed.). (2004b). *Using workbooks in mental health: Resources in prevention, psychotherapy, and rehabilitation for clinicians and researchers.* Binghamton, NY: Haworth.

L'Abate, L. (2005). *Personality in intimate relationships: Socialization and psychopathology.* New York: Springer-Science.

L'Abate, L. (Ed.). (2007c). *Low-cost approaches to promote physical and mental health: Theory, research, and practice.* New York: Springer-Science.

L'Abate, L. (2009a). A bibliography of secondary references for relational competence theory. In L. L'Abate, P. De Giacomo, M. Capitelli, & S. Longo (Eds.), *Science, mind, and creativity: The Bari Symposium* (pp. 175-196). Hauppauge, NY: Nova Science Publishers.

L'Abate, L. (2009b). A historical and systematic perspective about distance writing and wellness. In J. F. Evans (Ed.), *Wellness & writing connections: Writing for better physical, mental, and spiritual health* (pp. 53-74). Enumclaw, WA: Idyll Arbor, Inc.

L'Abate, L. (2009c). In search of a relational theory. *American Psychologist, 64,* 776-788.

L'Abate, L. (2011a). *Hurt feelings: Theory, research, and applications in intimate relationships.* New York: Cambridge University Press.

L'Abate, L. (2011b). Psychotherapy consists of homework assignments: A radical iconoclastic conviction. In H. Rosenthal (Ed.), *Favorite counseling and therapy homework techniques: Classic Anniversary Edition* (pp. 219-229). New York: Routledge.

L'Abate, L. (2011c). *Sourcebook of practice exercises in mental health.* New York: Springer-Science.

L'Abate, L. (2012). Workbooks: Programmed interactive practice exercises. In L. L'Abate & D. A. Kaiser (Eds.), *Handbook of technology in psychology, psychiatry, and neurology: Theory, research, and practice* (pp. 000-000). New York: Nova Science Publishers.

L'Abate, L., & Cusinato, M. (2007). Linking theory with practice: Theory-derived interventions in prevention and psychotherapy. *The Family Journal: Counseling and Therapy for Couples and Families, 15,* 318-327.

L'Abate, L., & Cusinato, M. (2008). Selfhood: A hidden ingredient in family therapy. *Journal of Family Psychotherapy*, 19, 320-329.

L'Abate, L., Cusinato, M., Maino, E., Colesso, W., & Scilletta, C. (2010). *Relational competence theory: Research and applications*. New York: Springer-Science

L'Abate, L., & De Giacomo, P. (2003). *Intimate relationships and how to improve them: Integrating theoretical models with preventive and psychotherapeutic applications*. Westport, CT: Praeger.

L'Abate, L., & Goldstein, D. (2007). Workbooks to promote mental health and life-long learning. In L. L'Abate (Ed.), *Low-cost interventions to promote physical and mental health: Theory, research and practice* (pp. 285-302). New York: Springer.

L'Abate, L., L'Abate, B. L., & Maino, E. (2005). A review of 25 years of part-time professional practice: Workbooks and length of psychotherapy. *American Journal of Family Therapy*, 33, 19-31.

L'Abate, L., & Sweeney, L. G. (Eds.). (2011). *Research on writing approaches in mental health*. Bingley, UK: Emerald Publishing Group Limited.

Lepore, S. J., & Smyth, J. M. (Eds.). (2002). *The writing cure: How expressive writing promotes health and emotional well-being*. Washington, DC: American Psychological Association.

Madden, G. J., & Bickel, W. K. (Eds.). (2010). *Impulsivity: The behavioral and neurological science of discounting*. Washington, DC: American Psychological Association.

Mansell, W. (2005). Control theory and psychopathology: An integrative approach. *Psychology and Psycho-therapy: Theory, Research, and Practice*, 78, 141-178.

Markon, K. E., Krueger, R. F., & Watson, D. (2005). Delineating the structure of normal and abnormal personality: An integrative hierarchical approach. *Journal of Personality and Social Psychology*, 88, 139-157.

Massel, H. K., Liberman, R. P., Mintz, J., Jacobs, H. E., et al. (1990). Evaluating the capacity to work in the mentally ill. *Psychiatry: Journal for the Study of Interpersonal Processes*, 53, 31-43.

McAdams, D. P. (1988). *Power, intimacy, and the life-story: Personological inquiries into identity*. New York: Guildford.

McHugh, P., & Slavney, P. (1989). *The perspectives of psychiatry*. Baltimore, MD: Johns Hopkins University Press.

Metts, S., & Grohskopf, E. (2003). Impression management: Goals, strategies, and skills. In J. O. Greene B. R. Burleson (Eds.), *Handbook of communication and social interaction skills* (pp. 357-399). Mahwah, NJ: Erlbaum.

Mikulincer, M., & Shaver, P. R. (2007). *Adult attachment: Structure, dynamics, and change*. New York: Guilford.

Millon T., Blaney, P. H, & Davis, R. D. (Eds.). (1999). *Oxford textbook of psycho-pathology*. New York: Oxford University Press.

Morry, M. M., (2005). Relationship satisfaction as a predictor of similarity ratings: A test of the similarity-attraction hypothesis. *Journal of Social and Personal Relationships*, 22, 561-584.

Nigg, J. T., Carr, L., Martel, M., & Henderson, J. M. (2007). Concepts of inhibition and developmental psychopathology. In D. S. Gorfein& C. M. MacLeod (Eds.), *Inhibition in cognition* (pp. 259-277). Washington, DC: American Psychological Association.

Omer, H. (1985). Fulfillment of therapeutic tasks as a precondition for acceptance in therapy. *American Journal of Psychotherapy, 56,* 496-501.

Roloff, M. E., Putman, L. L., &Anastasiou, L. (2003). Negotiation skills. In J. O. Greene & B. R. Burleson (Eds.), *Handbook of communication and social interaction skills* (pp. 801-833). Mahwah, NJ: Erlbaum.

Smyth, J. M., & L'Abate, L. (2001). A meta-analytic evaluation of workbook effectiveness in physical and mental health. In L. L'Abate (Ed.), *Distance writing and computer-assisted interventions in psychiatry and mental health* (pp.77-90). Westport, CT: Ablex.

Permissions

The contributors of this book come from diverse backgrounds, making this book a truly international effort. This book will bring forth new frontiers with its revolutionizing research information and detailed analysis of the nascent developments around the world.

We would like to thank Prof. Dr. Luciano L'Abate, for lending his expertise to make the book truly unique. He has played a crucial role in the development of this book. Without his invaluable contribution this book wouldn't have been possible. He has made vital efforts to compile up to date information on the varied aspects of this subject to make this book a valuable addition to the collection of many professionals and students.

This book was conceptualized with the vision of imparting up-to-date information and advanced data in this field. To ensure the same, a matchless editorial board was set up. Every individual on the board went through rigorous rounds of assessment to prove their worth. After which they invested a large part of their time researching and compiling the most relevant data for our readers. Conferences and sessions were held from time to time between the editorial board and the contributing authors to present the data in the most comprehensible form. The editorial team has worked tirelessly to provide valuable and valid information to help people across the globe.

Every chapter published in this book has been scrutinized by our experts. Their significance has been extensively debated. The topics covered herein carry significant findings which will fuel the growth of the discipline. They may even be implemented as practical applications or may be referred to as a beginning point for another development. Chapters in this book were first published by InTech; hereby published with permission under the Creative Commons Attribution License or equivalent.

The editorial board has been involved in producing this book since its inception. They have spent rigorous hours researching and exploring the diverse topics which have resulted in the successful publishing of this book. They have passed on their knowledge of decades through this book. To expedite this challenging task, the publisher supported the team at every step. A small team of assistant editors was also appointed to further simplify the editing procedure and attain best results for the readers.

Our editorial team has been hand-picked from every corner of the world. Their multi-ethnicity adds dynamic inputs to the discussions which result in innovative outcomes. These outcomes are then further discussed with the researchers and contributors who give their valuable feedback and opinion regarding the same. The feedback is then collaborated with the researches and they are edited in a comprehensive manner to aid the understanding of the subject.

Apart from the editorial board, the designing team has also invested a significant amount of their time in understanding the subject and creating the most relevant covers. They scrutinized every image to scout for the most suitable representation of the subject and create an appropriate cover for the book.

The publishing team has been involved in this book since its early stages. They were actively engaged in every process, be it collecting the data, connecting with the contributors or procuring relevant information. The team has been an ardent support to the editorial, designing and production team. Their endless efforts to recruit the best for this project, has resulted in the accomplishment of this book. They are a veteran in the field of academics and their pool of knowledge is as vast as their experience in printing. Their expertise and guidance has proved useful at every step. Their uncompromising quality standards have made this book an exceptional effort. Their encouragement from time to time has been an inspiration for everyone.

The publisher and the editorial board hope that this book will prove to be a valuable piece of knowledge for researchers, students, practitioners and scholars across the globe.

List of Contributors

Zikrija Dostović, Dževdet Smajlović and Omer Ć. Ibrahimagić
Department of Neurology, University Clinical Center Tuzla, School of Medicine, University of Tuzla, Bosnia and Herzegovina

Ernestina Dostović
Department of Anaesthesiology and Reanimatology, University Clinical Center Tuzla, School of Medicine, University of Tuzla, Bosnia and Herzegovina

Mary Ditton
University of New England, Australia

Maja Rus-Makovec
University Psychiatric Hospital Ljubljana & School of Medicine, University of Ljubljana, Slovenia

Charl Els, Diane Kunyk, Harold Hoffman and Adam Wargon
University of Alberta, Canada

Mamdouh El-Adl
Queen University, Kingston, Ontario, Canada

Yang Wang
Department of Psychiatry, School of Medicine Shandong University, Psychiatric Department, Shandong Mental Health Center, China

Mónica Figueira, Inmaculada Fuentes and Juan C. Ruiz
Faculty of Psychology, University of Valencia, Spain

Adeyi A. Adoga
Senior Lecturer/Consultant Ear, Nose, Throat, Head and Neck Surgeon, Department of Ear, Nose, Throat/ Head and Neck Surgery, University of Jos and Jos University Teaching Hospital, Nigeria

Luciano L'Abate
Georgia State University, USA

Mario Cusinato
University of Padova, Italy